Critical Issues in Health

Second Edition

Dr. Lana Zinger

Queensborough Community College

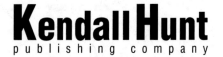

D1444424

Previously titled: *Health for Life: A Comprehensive Guide to Health and Wellness*

Cover and chapter opener images © Shutterstock, Inc.

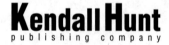

www.kendallhunt.com
Send all inquires to:
4050 Westmark Drive
Dubuque, IA 52004-1840

Printed in the United States of America
10 9 8 7 6 5 4 3 2 1

....

Health, the greatest of all we count as blessings.
—Ariphron

....

**I count my blessings every day thanks to my two highly
energetic and spirited boys, Max and Alexander.**

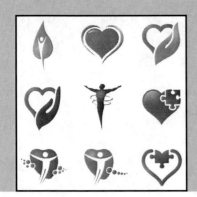

Contents

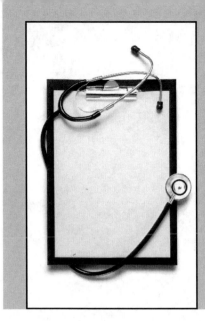

Chapter 1

Overview
of Health

How Healthy Are You?

1. How much extra weight are you carrying around (be honest)?
   - None at all
   - I have a few extra pounds
   - More than 10 pounds
   - I am seriously overweight
2. How much regular exercise do you get?
   - None at all
   - A few times per week
   - Almost every day
3. How much TV/Internet time do you spend a day?
   - None
   - 1–2 hours
   - 3–5 hours
   - 6–8 hours
   - 8+ hours
4. How many meals do you eat per day?
   - 1
   - 2
   - 3
   - More than 3

5. How often do you eat fast food?
   - Never
   - Maybe once per month
   - A couple times per month
   - A few times per week
   - Virtually every day

6. How often do you eat whole grains, oats, cereal and wholegrain bread?
   - Never
   - Maybe once per month
   - A couple times per month
   - A few times per week
   - Virtually every day

7. How many servings of fruit and vegetables do you eat each a day?
   - 5+
   - 3, 4
   - 1, 2
   - Virtually never

8. Do you watch your salt intake?
   - Never
   - Yes, I read food labels
   - I don't use any added salt

9. Apart from coffee or tea, what do you usually drink during the day?
   - Water
   - Soda/diet soda
   - Fruit juice
   - Sports drinks

10. Do you take a daily vitamin?
   - Every day
   - Most days
   - Some days
   - Never

11. Are you a smoker?
   - Not at all, never was
   - No, I quit
   - I am a social smoker
   - A few cigarettes per day
   - At least one pack per day

12. Do you live or work with a smoker?
   - Yes
   - No

13. How much alcohol do you drink per week?
    - None at all
    - A few drinks per week
    - I drink heavily a few times per week
    - I have a few drinks every day
    - I drink pretty heavily every day
14. Do you use "recreational" drugs?
    - Never
    - From time to time
    - Probably once a week
    - Very regularly
15. What is your level of school stress?
    - None really
    - A little bit here and there
    - I have pretty regular stress at school
    - Almost every minute of the day at school is stressful for me
16. What is your level of home stress?
    - None really
    - A little bit here and there
    - I have pretty regular stress at home
    - Almost every minute of the day at home is stressful for me
17. What is your outlook on life?
    - I have a very happy disposition
    - I'm a cautious optimist
    - I am skeptical about a lot of stuff
    - I require a lot of evidence but then I embrace good things
    - I think the world is pretty much all crap all the time
18. Do you have any family history of heart disease?
    - Yes
    - No
19. Has anyone in your immediate family suffered a stroke before the age of 50?
    - Yes
    - No
20. Has anyone in your family been diagnosed with cancer?
    - Yes
    - No
21. Has anyone in your family been diagnosed with diabetes?
    - Yes
    - No
22. Based on the above answers, do you think you are healthy?
    - Yes
    - No

23. Why or why not?

_____

_____

_____

_____

_____

24. Which area(s) if any, do you think you should work on improving?

_____

_____

_____

_____

_____

25. Name the most important health concerns facing you, your community, family, and/or friends:

_____

_____

_____

_____

_____

Definitions of Health and Wellness

Health is a subjective concept that is defined in relationship to cultural values and social norms. The World Health Organization defines health as being sound in body, mind, and spirit. It is not merely the absence of disease or infirmity, but a state of complete physical, mental, and social well-being.[1] A Report of the Surgeon General states that health means being physically fit enough to have mental functions of thinking, reasoning, feeling, and thoughts about purposive behavior.[2] Similarly, wellness is defined as a deliberate lifestyle choice characterized by personal responsibility and optimal enhancement of physical, mental, and spiritual health.

Components of Health

1. Physical—nutrition (food/weight/BMI)
2. Emotional—expression and control of emotions; self-esteem
3. Environmental—appreciation of external environment and your role in improving and protecting your surroundings
4. Intellectual—ability to think, analyze, and use brain power successfully and effectively in dealing with situations
5. Spiritual—hopes for life; what your existence means
6. Social—interactions with others

Life Expectancy

The average number of years a newborn is expected to live with current mortality patterns remaining the same.

> United States = 78.4 years of age

As of September 23, 2010, the United States currently ranks 49th in the world in overall life expectancy, according to a study published in the Journal of Health Affairs, slipping dramatically during the last decade. The decline is highlighted by the fact that in 1999, the World Health Organization ranked the U.S. as 24th in the world in life expectancy. Obesity, smoking, traffic fatalities, and homicide are strong reasons for this low rank, but a recent study zoned in on flaws in the nation's health-care system as the main culprit.

The study, "What Changes in Survival Rates Tell Us about U.S. Health Care," which was funded by the Commonwealth Fund, found that failings in the U.S. health care system, such as costly specialized and fragmented care, are likely playing a large role in this relatively poor performance on improvements in life expectancy. The United States spends over twice as much per capita on health care than other industrialized nations, so why do we have shorter life expectancies?

All the focus is on profit instead of focusing on preventive care, wellness, healthy food and water, and a safe environment.

Factors for Increased Life Expectancy

- Vaccinations
- Control of infectious diseases
- Fluoridation of drinking water
- Pasteurization of milk
- Safer storage of food
- Safer workplaces
- Motor vehicle safety

Top 10 Leading Causes of Death for All Ages in the United States[3]

1. Heart disease
2. Cancer
3. Stroke
4. Lung disease

5. Diabetes
6. Influenza/pneumonia
7. Alzheimer's disease
8. Motor vehicle (MV) crashes
9. Kidney disease
10. Septicemia (systemic blood infection)

Top 10 Leading Causes of Death for Young Adults in the United States[4]

1. MV crashes
2. Homicide
3. Suicide
4. Accidental poisoning
5. Cancer
6. Heart disease
7. Accidental drowning
8. Congenital abnormalities
9. Accidental falls
10. HIV/AIDS

The Centers for Disease Control and Prevention's (CDC) Six Critical Health Behaviors:

1. **Tobacco use** remains the leading preventable cause of death in the United States. Each year cigarette smoking accounts for approximately 1 of every 5 deaths, or about 400,000 people. Each day in the United States, approximately 3,600 young people between the ages of 12 and 17 years start cigarette smoking. In 2009, 19% of high schools students reported current cigarette use and 14% reported current cigar use. In addition, 9% of high school students and 20% of white male high school students reported current smokeless tobacco use.

2. **Unhealthy eating** is associated with increased risk for many diseases, including the three leading causes of death: heart disease, cancer, and stroke. In 2009, only 22.3% of high school students reported eating fruits and vegetables five or more times during the past 7 days.

3. **Inadequate physical activity** increases the risk of premature death and diseases such as heart disease, hypertension, cancer, and diabetes. Regular physical activity in childhood and adolescence improves academic performance, especially memory retention, strength and endurance, helps build healthy bones and muscles, helps control weight, reduces anxiety and stress, increases self-esteem, and improves blood pressure and cholesterol levels. The U.S. Department of Health and Human Services recommends that young people participate in at least 60 minutes of physical activity *daily*. In 2009, 18% of high school students had participated in at least 60 minutes per day of physical and only 33% attended physical education class daily.

4. **Unsafe sexual behaviors.** Vaginal, anal, and oral intercourse place young people at risk for HIV infection and other sexually transmitted diseases (STDs). In 2009, 46% of high school students had ever had sexual intercourse, and 14% of high school students had had four or more sex partners during their life. 34% of sexually active high school students did not use a condom. 22% of high school students who had sexual intercourse during the past three months drank alcohol or used drugs before last sexual intercourse.

5. **Alcohol and drug use**
   - Alcohol is one of the most widely used drug substances in the world. Alcohol is used by more young people in the United States than tobacco or illicit drugs. Excessive alcohol consumption is associated with approximately 75,000 deaths per year.
   - Long-term alcohol misuse is associated with liver disease, cancer, cardiovascular disease, and neurological damage as well as psychiatric problems such as depression, anxiety, and antisocial personality disorder.
   - Marijuana is the most commonly used illicit drug among youth in the United States.
   - Prescription and over-the-counter drug abuse remain high. Prescription medications most commonly abused by youth include pain relievers, tranquilizers, stimulants, and depressants. In 2009, 20% of U.S. high school students reported taking a prescription drug, such as Oxycontin, Percocet, Vicodin, Adderall, Ritalin, or Xanax, without a doctor's prescription. Teens also misuse OTC cough and cold medications containing the cough suppressant dextromethorphan (DXM), such as Robitussin, to get high.

6. **Injury and violence** are the leading cause of death and disability for people aged 1 to 44 years. Approximately 72% of all deaths among adolescents aged 10–24 years are attributed to injuries from four causes: motor vehicle crashes (30%), all other unintentional injuries (15%), homicide (15%), and suicide (12%). Highly associated with these injuries are adolescent behaviors such as physical fights, carrying weapons, making a suicide plan, and not using seatbelts.

Healthy People 2010

What Are the Leading Health Indicators?

The Leading Health Indicators will be used to measure the health of the nation over the next 10 years. Each of the 10 Leading Health Indicators has one or more objectives from Healthy People 2010 associated with it. As a group, the Leading Health Indicators reflect the major health concerns in the United States at the beginning of the 21st century. The Leading Health Indicators were selected on the basis of their ability to motivate action, the availability of data to measure progress, and their importance as public health issues.

The Leading Health Indicators are:

- Physical Activity
- Overweight and Obesity
- Tobacco Use
- Substance Abuse
- Responsible Sexual Behavior
- Mental Health
- Injury and Violence
- Environmental Quality
- Immunization
- Access to Health Care

- Healthy People 2010[5] is a federal initiative for health promotion and disease prevention for the nation.
- Every decade the federal government identifies the most significant preventable threats to health and creates leading indicators that assess the health of Americans.
- Healthy People 2010 has more than 450 health objectives organized into 28 areas and two overarching goals:

Goal 1
- To help individuals of all ages increase life expectancy and improve their quality of life.

Goal 2
- To eliminate health disparities among different segments of the population.

How do you propose to achieve goals 1 and 2?

_____

_____

_____

_____

_____

_____

_____

Achieving Goal 1
- Increase the number of adolescents engaging in physical activity of at least 20 minutes duration for a minimum of three days per week.
- Increase the number of adults engaging in physical activity for at least 30 minutes three days per week.
- Reduce obesity rates in children and adults.
- Reduce the percentage of teens and adults who smoke.
- Reduce the percentage of teens and adults who use illegal substances.
- Reduce the percentage of teens and adults who binge drink.
- Increase the percentage of responsible sexual behavior.

Achieving Goal 2
- Provide health insurance for all.
- Increase access to health care.
- Decrease poverty, discrimination, and illegal immigration status.
- Increase income and minimum wage.

Can Race Affect Health?
- The infant mortality rate is higher for African Americans.[6]
- Life expectancy is lower for African Americans.[7]

- African Americans have higher rates of hypertension.
- Native Americans have the highest diabetes rates.
- Caucasians have higher rates of osteoporosis, cystic fibrosis, skin cancer, and phenylketonuria (PKU).
- Chinese and Latina women have an increased risk of developing gestational diabetes.
- Asians metabolize some medications faster than whites.
- Ashkenazi Jews have higher rates of Tay-Sachs disease.[8]
- One in three Hispanics under the age of 65 has no health insurance.[9]

Factors Affecting Race and Health

- Genetics
- Environment
- Poverty
- Language barriers
- Unhealthy lifestyle
- Stress
- Illegal immigration status
- Income
- Education
- Discrimination

Can Gender Affect Health?[10]

- Women live longer than men.
- Women have higher rates of depression, panic attacks, arthritis, osteoporosis, and Alzheimer's disease.
- Women have higher rates of chronic diseases.
- Women score better on tests of verbal fluency.
- Women are more likely to be infected with a sexually transmitted disease (STD) during heterosexual contact.
- Women have a lower percentage of muscle.
- Women are more likely to attempt suicide.
- Men have higher rates of succeeding at suicide.
- Men are more prone to deadly diseases before age 50.
- Men suffer more injuries.
- Men score better in tests of visual-spatial ability.
- Men have higher rates of smoking and alcohol abuse.

How Healthy Is the U.S.?

- **Morbidity**—The relative incidence of disease.
- **Mortality**—The proportion of deaths to population.

During the 1900s, communicable diseases accounted for about 60 percent of all deaths. The top three causes of death in the United States in 1900 were:

1. Pneumonia/influenza,
2. Tuberculosis, and
3. Diarrhea/enteritis

These diseases were eradicated or nearly eliminated through better living conditions, hygiene, and the invention of antibiotics and vaccines. However, changes in living brought in other diseases, including lifestyle diseases. Since the 1940s, most deaths in the United States have resulted from lifestyle diseases such as heart disease, cancer, and strokes. And, by the late 1990s, lifestyle diseases accounted for more than 60 percent of all deaths. Certain forms of cancer, heart disease, high blood pressure, obesity, and Type 2 diabetes are lifestyle diseases because they are contracted from the way people live. Poor diet, lack of exercise, smoking, and excess alcohol and drug use, and poor sleep may contribute to these illnesses or be their primary cause. Researchers are saying that today's newborns may be the first generation to have a lower life expectancy than that of their parents. This is due to lifestyle risk factors, specifically obesity.

Examples of lifestyle diseases:

- Heart disease, "the #1 killer of both women and men," according to the National Institutes of Health, is most often caused by being overweight, not exercising, and smoking.

- Type 2 diabetes is when your body does not produce enough insulin or cannot use the insulin efficiently enough. This results in high blood sugar, since insulin is responsible for breaking down sugar to use for energy in the body. Diabetes can lead to long-term complications like kidney disease, blindness, and poor wound healing. The lifestyle risk factors for diabetes include being overweight, not eating a healthy diet and physical inactivity.

- Among the most common infectious diseases are those that are sexually transmitted, with the Centers for Disease Control and Prevention reporting "19 million new STD infections each year . . ." Not using condoms is a lifestyle decision that predisposes one to fall victim to an STD or HIV/AIDS.

Though people are predisposed to many chronic illnesses because of genetics, age, gender or race, there are lifestyle changes you can make to decrease your chances of being affected. A person's health is his most precious asset. Good health allows you to fully participate in work and social activities. Your abilities become severely impaired when disease enters your life, whether it is for a short time or over an indefinite period. While anyone can become ill, there are strategies you can employ to help prevent disease. These include lifestyle changes geared toward protecting your health.

We are what we repeatedly do. Excellence, then, is not an act, but a habit.
—Aristotle

Habits and Your Health

A habit is an automatic behavior. The behavior has become automatic because it has been repeated frequently and thereby, turned over to subconscious control. We are all forming and reinforcing habits every day of our lives. Some are positive habits that move us toward our goals and some are negative that move us away from our goals. Any behavior that you repeat every day is habit-forming!

List your positive habits:

_____

_____

_____

_____

List your negative habits:

_____

_____

_____

_____

Most Harmful Personal Habits

1. Smoking
2. Drinking too much alcohol
3. Spending yourself into deep debt
4. Needing sleeping pills to get a good night's sleep
5. Taking painkillers every day

Most Harmful Lifestyle Choices

1. Being angry, worried, or stressed more than being happy
2. Not feeling in control
3. Being in an unhealthy relationship
4. Ignoring health signs and symptoms of disease
5. Not moving your body every day

Most Harmful Eating Habits

1. Drinking a lot of soda
2. Eating fast food more than 3 days/week
3. Skipping breakfast
4. Not eating vegetables daily
5. Yo-yo dieting

The Power of Positive Habits:
How to Change a Habit

1. Health Belief Model

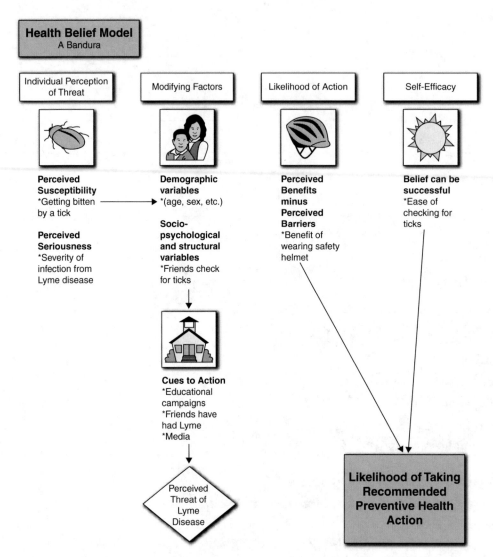

Health Belief Model
A Bandura

Individual Perception of Threat

Modifying Factors

Likelihood of Action

Self-Efficacy

Perceived Susceptibility
*Getting bitten by a tick

Perceived Seriousness
*Severity of infection from Lyme disease

Demographic variables
*(age, sex, etc.)

Socio-psychological and structural variables
*Friends check for ticks

Cues to Action
*Educational campaigns
*Friends have had Lyme
*Media

Perceived Threat of Lyme Disease

Perceived Benefits minus Perceived Barriers
*Benefit of wearing safety helmet

Belief can be successful
*Ease of checking for ticks

Likelihood of Taking Recommended Preventive Health Action

Source: Melanie Zibit MS, MBA, Medical Educator and Illustrator, Nancy Shadick, MD, MPH, and Brigham & Women's Hospital. Reproduced with permission.

The Health Belief Model (HBM) is a psychological model that attempts to explain and predict health behaviors. This is done by focusing on the attitudes and beliefs of individuals. The HBM was first developed in the 1950s by social psychologists Hochbaum, Rosenstock and Kegels working in the U.S. Public Health Services. The model was inspired by a study of why people sought X-ray examinations for tuberculosis. Since then, the HBM has been adapted to explore a variety of long- and short-term health behaviors, including sexual risk behaviors and the transmission of HIV/AIDS. The model postulates that the following six conditions both explain and predict a health-related behavior.

1. **Perceived Susceptibility**. A person believes that his or her health is in jeopardy. People will not change their health behaviors unless they believe that they are at risk. *Those who do not think that they are at risk of acquiring HIV from unprotected intercourse are unlikely to use a condom.*

2. **Perceived Severity**. The probability that a person will change his/her health behaviors to avoid a consequence depend on how serious he or she considers the consequence to be. The person perceives the "potential seriousness" of the condition in terms of pain or discomfort, time lost from work, economic difficulties, or other outcomes.

3. **Perceived Benefits**. It's difficult to convince people to change a behavior if there isn't something in it for them. *Your father stopped smoking because the doctor said his lungs are failing.* On assessing the circumstances, the person believes that benefits stemming from the recommended behavior outweigh the costs and inconvenience and that they are indeed possible and within his or her grasp.

4. **Perceived Barriers**. One of the major reasons people don't change their health behaviors is that they think that doing so is going to be hard. Changing your health behaviors can cost effort, money, and time. *If all your friends go out drinking on Saturdays, it may be very difficult to cut down on your alcohol intake.*

5. **Cues to Action**. External events that prompt a desire to make a health change. A cue to action is something that helps move someone from wanting to make a health change to actually making the change.

6. **Self-efficacy**. Looks at a person's belief in his/her ability to make a health related change. The belief in your ability to do something has an enormous impact on your actual ability to do it. Thinking that you will fail will almost make certain that you do.

From *Encyclopedia of Public Health* edited by Lester Breslow. Copyright © 2002 by MacMillan Reference USA.

2. Stages of Change Model

Anyone who has ever made and broken a New Year's Resolution can appreciate the difficulty of behavior change. Making a lasting change in behavior is rarely a simple process, and usually involves a substantial commitment of time, effort, and emotion. The Stages of Change Model was originally developed in the late 1970s and early 1980s by James Prochaska and Carlo DiClemente at the University of Rhode Island when they were studying how smokers were able to give up their habits or addiction.

Stage 1: Precontemplation

When you're at this stage, you aren't even admitting you have a problem. Precontemplators don't want to change themselves. They think others are to blame for their difficulties. Smokers who are "in denial" may not see that the advice applies to them personally. Patients with high cholesterol levels may feel "immune" to the health problems that strike others. Obese patients may have tried unsuccessfully so many times to lose weight that they have simply given up.

Stage 2: Contemplation

In this stage, you acknowledge you have a problem. You begin to think seriously about solving your problem. You start to assess barriers (e.g., time, expense, hassle, fear,) as well as the benefits of change. You have indefinite plans to take action within the next few months.

Stage 3: Preparation

"If you fail to plan, you plan to fail."

You develop a detailed plan of action. You might be sampling low-fat foods or a move toward greater dietary modification, or decreasing your drinking.

Stage 4: Action

This stage is where you actually DO IT! You receive the most recognition and support during this stage, because others can see that you're working at it. You follow the plan you've made in Stage 3, making revisions as necessary.

Stage 5: Maintenance

The maintenance stage is a long, ongoing process, and for most people, it's the most difficult.

Celebrate achieving your goals, but don't relax just yet. Develop mental and behavioral coping strategies that will take you through the times when you feel you are beginning to slip.

Stage 6: Relapse

You must always maintain a life of vigilance. Some can progress to the point that they are not constantly tempted, nor do they think about it every day. Once you've had a deeply ingrained habit or addiction, you are always more vulnerable than if you'd never had it. Studies show that in times of stress or conflict, people are most likely to slip.

. . . .

> Habit is habit, and not to be flung out of the window by any man,
> but coaxed downstairs a step at a time.
>
> —*Mark Twain*

. . . .

Steps to Change Unhealthy Behaviors

1. **Work on one habit at a time**. If you work on changing more than one habit at a time you run a serious risk of overwhelming yourself and changing no habits at all. To begin with, choose one unhealthy habit you wish to eliminate or change. Or, choose a healthy habit you want to adopt as part of your behavior. **It takes 21–30 days to break a bad habit**.

2. **Start small**. The smaller the better, because habit change is difficult, and trying to take on too much is a recipe for disaster. Want to exercise? Start with just 10–20 minutes.

3. **Create a plan and write it down**. Be as specific as possible. **Refine** your plan. Now you need to refine your plan. In particular, you need to be realistic. Put your plan in a drawer for a day or so and come back to it with fresh eyes. Make Mini-Plans (research psychologists call them 'implementation intentions'). Write down all the details to make your big plan successful. For example, "when the alarm goes off at five, I will shower, get dressed, make a breakfast shake, and drive to work then at 5:30, I will eat a quick snack of yogurt and fruit and go to the gym." Researchers have shown the power of mini-plans to bridge the gap between wanting to get something done and getting it done. **Plan a support system**. Who will you turn to when you have a strong urge? Write these people into your plan. **Have rewards**. You might see these as bribes, but actually they're just positive feedback.

4. **Know your motivations, and be sure they're strong**. Write them down in your plan. You have to be very clear why you're doing this, and what the benefits are.

5. **Write down all your obstacles**. Write down every obstacle that's likely to happen. Then write down how you plan to overcome them. That's the key: write down your solution *before* the obstacles arrive, so you're prepared.

6. **Identify your triggers**. What situations trigger your current habit? For the smoking habit, for example, triggers might include going out with friends . . .

7. **For every single trigger, identify a positive habit you're going to do instead**. What will you do when you go out with friends, instead of smoking? What if someone offers you a cigarette? Some positive habits could include: exercise, meditation, deep breathing, and visualization.

8. **Become aware of self-talk**. Negative thoughts can derail any habit change. "I can't do this. This is too difficult. Why am I putting myself through this? How bad is this for me anyway?" It's important to take these negative thoughts and push them out of your head. Then replace them with a positive thought. "I can do this!"

9. **Plan strategies to defeat the negative urges**. Urges are going to come and go and they can be very strong and persuasive. But they're also temporary, and beatable. Urges usually last a few minutes, and they come in waves. You just need to ride out the wave, and the urge will go away. Some strategies for making it through the urge: deep breathing, self-massage, eat some frozen grapes, take a walk, exercise, drink a glass of water, call a support buddy, distract yourself.

10. **Use visualization**. This is a powerful tool. Vividly picture, in your head, successfully changing your habit. Visualize doing your new habit after each trigger, overcoming urges, and what it will look like when you're done.

11. **If you fail, figure out what went wrong, plan for it, and try again**. Don't let failure and guilt stop you. They're just obstacles, but they can be overcome. You should learn from each failure, and then they will become stepping stones to your success. When you fall off the horse, you have to get back on.

What Can You Do to Improve Your Health?

- Wear a seat belt.
- Stop smoking, binge-drinking, and abusing drugs.
- Exercise.
- Cut down on fast food.
- Cut down on caffeine.
- Reach your ideal body weight.
- Drink eight glasses of water every day.
- Perform regular body self-exams.
- Take regular stress breaks.
- Get enough sleep.
- Eat your fruits and vegetables.
- Volunteer.
- Be kind to yourself and to others.

Determining Your Personal Goals

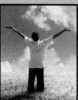

1. My personal goal is

_____

_____

_____

_____

_____

_____

2. My professional goal is

_____

_____

_____

_____

_____

_____

3. My social goal is

_____

_____

_____

_____

_____

_____

4. My psychological/emotional goal is

_____

_____

_____

_____

_____

_____

5. My spiritual goal is

_____

_____

_____

_____

_____

_____

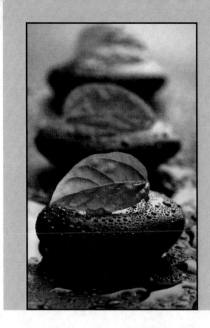

Chapter 2
Psychological Health

Are You Psychologically Healthy?

1. My sleep has become disturbed—too much, too little, or I wake up constantly.
   ○ Not at all   ○ Somewhat   ○ Quite a lot   ○ Nearly all the time

2. My mood swings from depression to happiness for no reason.
   ○ Not at all   ○ Somewhat   ○ Quite a lot   ○ Nearly all the time

3. I eat more than I should.
   ○ Not at all   ○ Somewhat   ○ Quite a lot   ○ Nearly all the time

4. I enjoy spending time playing a computer or online game more than I enjoy most everything else in my life.
   ○ Not at all   ○ Somewhat   ○ Quite a lot   ○ Nearly all the time

5. People sometimes think that I'm unstable or unreliable.
   ○ Not at all   ○ Somewhat   ○ Quite a lot   ○ Nearly all the time

6. I have poor self-esteem.
   ○ Not at all   ○ Somewhat   ○ Quite a lot   ○ Nearly all the time

7. I often feel that I don't play any useful part in life.
   ○ Not at all   ○ Somewhat   ○ Quite a lot   ○ Nearly all the time

8. I have thought about ending my life.
   ○ Not at all   ○ Somewhat   ○ Quite a lot   ○ Nearly all the time

9. Sometimes I am overwhelmed by distractions or thoughts that I can't seem to control.
   ○ Not at all   ○ Somewhat   ○ Quite a lot   ○ Nearly all the time

10. I often have disturbing dreams or recollections about something that happened in my life.
    ○ Not at all   ○ Somewhat   ○ Quite a lot   ○ Nearly all the time

11. I hate the way I look.
    ○ Not at all   ○ Somewhat   ○ Quite a lot   ○ Nearly all the time

12. I often cry or go into a rage for no reason.
    ○ Not at all   ○ Somewhat   ○ Quite a lot   ○ Nearly all the time

13. My feelings or behaviors are interfering with work, school, friendships, or my relationship.
   ○ Not at all   ○ Somewhat   ○ Quite a lot   ○ Nearly all the time

14. I feel unhappy, sad or worthless.
   ○ Not at all   ○ Somewhat   ○ Quite a lot   ○ Nearly all the time

15. I feel out of control.
   ○ Not at all   ○ Somewhat   ○ Quite a lot   ○ Nearly all the time

16. I often feel empty or that my life has little meaning.
   ○ Not at all   ○ Somewhat   ○ Quite a lot   ○ Nearly all the time

17. Do you ever see or hear things when no one else is around?
   ○ Not at all   ○ Somewhat   ○ Quite a lot   ○ Nearly all the time

18. Do you ever think so fast that when you talk your mouth can't keep up with your thoughts?
   ○ Not at all   ○ Somewhat   ○ Quite a lot   ○ Nearly all the time

19. Do you avoid making friends in case they try and make a fool of you?
   ○ Not at all   ○ Somewhat   ○ Quite a lot   ○ Nearly all the time

20. I am finding it more difficult to cope with things than usual.
   ○ Not at all   ○ Somewhat   ○ Quite a lot   ○ Nearly all the time

21. I am having trouble concentrating at work or school.
   ○ Not at all   ○ Somewhat   ○ Quite a lot   ○ Nearly all the time

22. Based on the above answers, do you think you are psychologically healthy? Why or why not?

_____

_____

_____

_____

_____

_____

23. What psychological areas need improvement in your life?

_____

_____

_____

_____

_____

_____

Definition of Psychological Health

If you aren't sick or do not have any disease, it doesn't mean you are healthy. According to the World Health Organization (WHO), health is a state of complete physical, mental, and social well-being and not merely the absence of disease or infirmity.

So are you psychologically feeling well right now?

_____

_____

_____

_____

_____

Dimensions of Psychological Health

- Mental
- Emotional
- Spiritual
- Cultural

How would you describe your level of self-esteem?

_____

_____

_____

_____

_____

Self-Esteem

- Belief and pride in ourselves
- Ability to maintain, and often regain, a positive view of one's self, no matter what
- External factors versus internal factors
- Allows us to try things we've failed at and take on new challenges

Boosting Self-Esteem

- Receive/provide unconditional love.
- Set realistic expectations.
- Provide positive affirmations.
- Give compliments and encouragement.

Managing Your Moods

- Bad moods affect us an average of three out of every 10 days.[11]
- Men often manage moods with distractions or drugs.
- Women use talking, crying, and food to manage bad moods.

Positive Ways to Banish a Bad Mood

- Figure out what made you upset and try to fix it.
- Exercise.
- Take your mind off the bad mood.
- Smile.
- Listen to music.

What do you do to banish a bad mood?

_____

_____

_____

_____

_____

_____

Describe the characteristics of a psychologically healthy person.

_____

_____

_____

_____

_____

_____

Factors Affecting Happiness

- Genetics
- Relationships
- Gender and race
- Life events
- Education and intelligence
- Age, health, and wealth

Best Predictors of Happiness

- High self-esteem
- Optimism
- Extroversion
- Supportive relationships
- Sense of being in control

Bottom line: Feeling good does not necessarily depend on money, success, recognition, or status. Instead:

- Accept yourself.
- Respect yourself.
- Trust yourself.
- Love yourself.

What is the difference between everyday stressors and mental disorders?

According to the *Diagnostic and Statistical Manual of Mental Disorders (DSM-IV-TR)*, a mental disorder is a pattern of behavior in an individual that is associated with distress or disability or with significantly increased risk of suffering, death, pain, or loss of freedom. A mental disorder differs from everyday stressors or problems because a mental disorder can be diagnosed from a set of symptoms. Worries, fears, anxieties are common, especially during the college years. Most people gradually learn how to deal with life's problems through positive behavior change.

Mental Disorders

Mental disorders include diagnosable mental, behavioral, or emotional disorders that interfere with one or more major activities. One of every two Americans who need mental health treatment do not receive it, and the rate is even lower—and the quality of care poorer—for ethnic and racial minorities.

Panic Attacks

Panic disorder is characterized by unexpected and repeated episodes of intense fear accompanied by physical symptoms that may include chest pain, heart palpitations, shortness of breath, dizziness, or abdominal distress. These sensations often mimic symptoms of a heart attack.

Occurrence

- In a given year 1.7 percent of the U.S. population (2.4 million Americans) experiences panic disorder.
- Women are twice as likely as men to develop panic disorder.
- Panic disorder typically strikes in young adulthood. Roughly half of all people who have panic disorder develop the condition before age 24.[12]

Causes

- Heredity
- Biological
- Catastrophic thinking

Treatment

- Cognitive behavioral therapy: breathing, counting backwards, distraction
- Medication

Anxiety Disorder

Generalized anxiety disorder (GAD) is characterized by six months or more of chronic, exaggerated worry and tension that is unfounded or much more severe than the normal anxiety most people experience. People with this disorder usually expect the worst; they worry excessively about money, health, family, or work, even when there are no signs of trouble. They are unable to relax and often suffer from insomnia. Many people with GAD also have physical symptoms, such as fatigue, trembling, muscle tension, headaches, irritability, or hot flashes.[13]

Occurrence

- About 2.8 percent of the U.S. population (4 million Americans) has GAD during a year's time.
- GAD most often strikes people in childhood or adolescence, but can begin in adulthood, too.
- GAD affects women more often than men.[14]

Causes

- Stress
- Biological

Treatment

- Cognitive behavioral therapy
- Medication
- National Institute of Mental Health (NIMH) Anxiety Information Line: 1-888-8ANXIETY (826-9438)
- NIMH Panic Information Line: 1-888-64PANIC (647-2642)

Obsessive-Compulsive Disorder (OCD)

Individuals with OCD suffer intensely from recurrent, unwanted thoughts (obsessions) or rituals (compulsions) that they feel they cannot control. Rituals such as handwashing, counting, checking, or cleaning are often performed in hopes of preventing obsessive thoughts or making them go away. Performing these rituals, however, provides only temporary relief, and not performing them markedly increases anxiety. Left untreated, obsessions and the need to perform rituals can take over a person's life. OCD is often a chronic, relapsing illness.[15]

Occurrence

- About 2.3 percent of the U.S. population (3.3 million Americans) has OCD in a given year.
- OCD affects men and women equally.

- OCD typically begins during adolescence or early childhood; at least one-third of the cases of adult OCD began in childhood.
- OCD cost the United States $8.4 billion in 1990 in social and economic losses, nearly 6 percent of the total mental health bill of $148 billion.[16]

Causes
- Biological

Treatment
- Behavioral therapy
- Medications

Depression

Depression is the most common mental ailment in the world. Depression causes people to lose pleasure from daily life, can complicate other medical conditions, and can even be serious enough to lead to suicide. Depression is characterized as a sadness that does not end.

Symptoms
- Persistent sad, anxious or "empty" mood
- Sleeping too much or too little; middle of the night or early morning waking
- Reduced appetite and weight loss, or increased appetite and weight gain
- Loss of pleasure and interest in activities once enjoyed, including sex
- Restlessness, irritability
- Persistent physical symptoms that do not respond to treatment (such as chronic pain or digestive disorders)
- Difficulty concentrating, remembering, or making decisions
- Fatigue or loss of energy, feeling guilty, hopeless, or worthless
- Thoughts of suicide or death[17]

> *If you have five or more of these symptoms for two weeks or more, you could have clinical depression and should see your doctor or a qualified mental health professional for help.*

Occurrence
- Clinical depression is one of the most common mental illnesses, affecting more than 19 million Americans each year.[18]
- Depression can affect anyone, at any age, and people of any race or ethnic group.
- Teens born in the 1980s are more likely to develop depression than those who were born in the 1970s, whose rate of depression is higher than those born in the 1960s.[19]

Causes
- *Biological*—People with depression typically have too little or too much of certain brain chemicals, called *neurotransmitters*. Changes in these brain chemicals may cause or contribute to clinical depression.
- *Cognitive*—People with negative thinking patterns and low self-esteem are more likely to develop clinical depression.

- *Gender*—Women experience clinical depression at a rate that is nearly twice that of men. Though the reasons for this are still unclear, they may include the hormonal changes women go through during menstruation, pregnancy, childbirth, and menopause. Other reasons may include the stress caused by the multiple responsibilities that women have.
- *Co-occurrence*—Clinical depression is more likely to occur along with certain illnesses, such as heart disease, cancer, Parkinson's disease, diabetes, Alzheimer's disease, and hormonal disorders.
- *Medications*—Side effects of some medications can bring about depression.
- *Genetic*—A family history of clinical depression increases the risk for developing the illness.
- *Situational*—Difficult life events, including divorce, financial problems or the death of a loved one, can contribute to clinical depression.[20]

Treatment

- Psychotherapy
- Medication

Why do you think so many young people are depressed?

_____

_____

_____

_____

_____

_____

Tips for Dealing with Depression for College Students
- Carefully plan your day.
- Get enough sleep.
- Exercise.
- Participate in extracurricular activities.
- Seek support from other people.
- Try relaxation methods.
- Take time for yourself every day.
- Seek treatment, such as through a college counseling center.

Bipolar Disorder

Bipolar disorder, also known as manic depression, is an illness involving one or more episodes of serious mania and depression. The illness causes a person's mood to swing from excessively "high" and/or irritable to sad and hopeless, with periods of a normal mood in between. More than 2 million Americans suffer from bipolar disorder.

Symptoms

- Excessive energy, activity, restlessness, racing thoughts, and rapid talking
- Denial that anything is wrong
- Extreme "high" or euphoric feelings
- Easily irritated or distracted
- Decreased need for sleep
- Unrealistic beliefs in one's ability and powers
- Uncharacteristically poor judgment
- Sustained period of behavior that is different from usual
- Unusual sexual drive
- Abuse of drugs, particularly cocaine, alcohol, or sleeping medications
- Provocative, intrusive, or aggressive behavior[21]

Occurrence

- Typically begins in adolescence or early adulthood and continues throughout life

Causes

- Genetic
- Biochemical

Treatment

- Professional help
- Medication
- Support from family, friends, and peers

Suicide

Suicide is not a psychiatric disorder, but it is the consequence of psychological problems.

Occurrence

- Approximately 30,000 Americans commit suicide annually; an additional 752,000 Americans attempt suicide annually; there may be 4.5 million suicide survivors in the United States.[22]
- Women attempt more suicides, but men are more successful.
- Suicide is the third leading cause of death in young adults.

Warning Signs

- Verbal threats
- Expressions of hopelessness and helplessness
- Previous suicide attempts
- Daring or risk-taking behavior
- Personality changes
- Depression
- Giving away possessions
- Lack of interest in future plans

Factors That Protect Against Suicide

- Feeling connected to family and friends
- Emotional well-being
- Avoiding drugs and alcohol

What to do if you think someone is suicidal

- Trust your instincts that the person may be in trouble.
- Talk with the person about your concerns. Communication needs to include *listening*.
- Ask direct questions without being judgmental. Determine if the person has a specific plan to carry out the suicide. The more detailed the plan, the greater the risk.
- Get professional help, even if the person resists.
- Contact the hotline at 1-800-SUICIDE (1-800-784-2433) or www.hopeline.com. This will connect you with a crisis center in your area.
- Do not leave the person alone.
- Do not swear to secrecy.
- Do not act shocked or judgmental.
- Do not counsel the person yourself.[23]

Attention Deficit/Hyperactivity Disorder (ADHD)

Signs and Symptoms

- Impulsiveness
- Inattention
- Hyperactivity

Occurrence

- Three times as many boys as girls are affected by ADHD.[24]

Causes

- Genetic
- Biological
- Differences within the brain
- Prenatal use of tobacco, alcohol, or cocaine
- Delivery complications
- Postnatal illnesses

Treatment

- Behavioral therapy
- Medication

Schizophrenia

Someone with schizophrenia may have difficulty distinguishing between what is real and what is imaginary, may be unresponsive or withdrawn, and may have difficulty expressing normal emotions in social situations.

Signs and Symptoms

- Delusions—false ideas; individuals may believe that someone is spying on them, or that they are someone famous.
- Hallucinations—seeing, feeling, tasting, hearing, or smelling something that doesn't really exist. The most common experience is hearing imaginary voices that give commands or comments to the individual.
- Disordered thinking and speech—moving quickly from one topic to another, in a nonsensical fashion. Individuals may make up their own words or sounds.
- Social withdrawal
- Extreme apathy
- Lack of drive or initiative
- Emotional unresponsiveness[25]

Occurrence

- Mean age for development is 21.4 in men and 26.8 in women.[26]

Causes

- Genetics (heredity)
- Biology (imbalance in the brain's chemistry)
- Viral infections and immune disorders

Treatment

- No cure exists
- Antipsychotic medication
- Psychiatric counseling
- Housing programs
- Case management

Seasonal Affective Disorder (SAD)

Some people suffer from symptoms of depression during the winter months, with symptoms subsiding during the spring and summer months. As seasons change, there is a shift in our "biological internal clocks" or circadian rhythm, due partly to these changes in sunlight patterns. This can cause our biological clocks to be out of step with our daily schedules. The most difficult months for SAD sufferers are January and February, and younger persons and women are at higher risk.

Signs and Symptoms

- Regularly occurring symptoms of depression (excessive eating and sleeping, weight gain) during the fall or winter months.
- Full remission from depression in the spring and summer months.
- Symptoms have occurred in the past two years, with no nonseasonal depression episodes.
- Seasonal episodes substantially outnumber nonseasonal depression episodes.
- A craving for sugary and/or starchy foods.[27]

Causes

Melatonin, a sleep-related hormone secreted by the pineal gland in the brain, has been linked to SAD. This hormone, which may cause symptoms of depression, is produced at increased levels in the dark. Therefore, when the days are shorter and darker the production of this hormone increases.

Treatment

- Phototherapy or bright light therapy
- One hour's walk in winter sunlight
- Antidepressant drugs

Social Anxiety

Social Anxiety is characterized by overwhelming anxiety and excessive self-consciousness in everyday social situations.

Signs and Symptoms

- Persistent, intense, and chronic fear of being watched and judged by others
- Feeling embarrassment or humiliation over own actions
- Fear interferes with work or school or other ordinary activities
- Physical signs such as blushing, sweating, trembling, nausea, and difficulty talking[28]

Treatment

- Behavioral therapy
- Antidepressant therapy

Shyness

Shyness is a form of social anxiety, a fear of what others will think of one's behavior or appearance. Shy people are often excessively self-critical, and they engage in very negative self-talk. Shy people often long to be more outgoing, but their own negative thoughts prevent them from enjoying the social interaction they desire.

Signs and Symptoms

- Rapid heartbeat
- Nervous stomach
- Clammy hands
- Dry mouth or lump in throat
- Trembling muscles

Occurrence

- Approximately 40 to 50 percent of Americans describe themselves as shy.
- Approximately 7 to 13 percent of adults are so shy that their condition interferes seriously with work, school, daily life, or interpersonal relationships.[29]

Causes

- Inherited trait
- Culture and parenting styles
- Stressful events
- Isolation

Treatment

- Shyness classes
- Assertiveness training
- Public speaking
- Cognitive behavioral therapy
- Antidepressant drugs

Post-Traumatic Stress Disorder (PTSD)

PTSD is an anxiety disorder that can develop after exposure to a terrifying event or ordeal in which grave physical harm occurred or was threatened. Traumatic events that may trigger PTSD include violent personal assaults, natural or human-caused disasters, accidents, or military combat.

Signs and Symptoms

Re-experiencing symptoms:
- Flashbacks—reliving the trauma over and over, including physical symptoms like a racing heart or sweating
- Bad dreams
- Frightening thoughts

Avoidance symptoms:
- Staying away from places, events, or objects that are reminders of the experience
- Feeling emotionally numb
- Feeling strong guilt, depression, or worry
- Losing interest in activities that were enjoyable in the past
- Having trouble remembering the dangerous event

Hyperarousal symptoms:
- Being easily startled
- Feeling tense or "on edge"
- Having difficulty sleeping and/or having angry outbursts

Treatment

- Psychotherapy ("talk" therapy)
- Exposure therapy
- Medications

Cutting and Self-harm

Self-injury (self-harm, self-mutilation, cutting) can be defined as the attempt to deliberately cause harm to one's own body and the injury is usually severe enough to cause tissue damage. This is not a conscious attempt at suicide. These are often ways to express deep distress and cope with painful memories.

Signs and Symptoms

- Unexplained wounds
- Indications of depression
- Frequent "accidents"
- Changes in eating habits
- Covering up

Treatment

- Choose a social worker, trauma therapist, psychologist, or psychiatrist who is trained in dealing with self-injury.

What to do when you feel like cutting yourself or self-harming

- **Deal with anger.** Try running, dancing fast, screaming, punching a pillow, throwing something, or ripping something apart.
- **Cope with emotional numbness.** Squeeze ice cubes, hold a package of frozen food, take a very cold shower, or chew something with a very strong taste, like chili peppers, raw ginger root, or a grapefruit peel.
- **Calm yourself.** Take a bubble bath, do deep breathing, write in a journal, draw, or practice yoga.
- **See "blood."** You can draw a red ink line where you would usually cut yourself, in addition to the other suggestions above.

Models of Therapeutic Change

The Behavioral Model

The behavioral model focuses on what people do—their overt behavior—rather than on brain structures and chemistry or on thoughts and consciousness. This model regards psychological problems as bad habits. Behaviorists analyze behavior in terms of stimulus, response, and reinforcement. Behavioral therapy focuses on changing the behavior by adapting a new, healthier habit. This treatment mode also uses exposure therapy, in which the person is exposed to his or her fear.

The Biological Model

The biological model emphasizes that the mind's activity depends entirely on an organic structure, the brain, whose composition is genetically determined. It focuses on genetic evidence and chemicals in the brain that influence our moods and mental health.

Cognitive Model

The cognitive model emphasizes the effect of ideas on behavior and feeling. This model believes that behavior results from complicated attitudes, expectations, and motives rather than simple, immediate reinforcements. It focuses on changing the way a person thinks about the feared situation.

Pharmacological Therapy

Pharmacological theory is inspired by the biological model. The brain communicates with itself use of special chemicals called neurotransmitters, such as *serotonin* and *norepinephrine*. There is a st relation between the amount of these chemicals in the brain and a person's mood. If levels of these c cals get too low, people feel depressed. Doctors can elevate these brain chemicals with the use of drugs.

Antidepressants

- *Selective serotonin reuptake inhibitors* (SSRIs)—These drugs increase the brain's level of serotonin, thus improving mood. SSRIs have also been shown to be useful in the treatment of obsessive-compulsive disorder and some forms of severe shyness. SSRIs include the following:
    - citalopram (brand name: Celexa)
    - escitalopram (brand name: Lexapro)
    - fluoxetine (brand name: Prozac)
    - paroxetine (brand names: Paxil, Pexeva)
    - sertraline (brand name: Zoloft)

These drugs come with strong warnings regarding their use with children. Some of the side effects that can be caused by SSRIs include dry mouth, nausea, nervousness, insomnia, sexual problems, headaches, and self-destructive thoughts.

- *Tricyclic antidepressants* get their name from their chemical structure:
    - amitriptyline (brand name: Elavil)
    - desipramine (brand name: Norpramin)
    - imipramine (brand name: Tofranil)
    - nortriptyline (brand name: Aventyl, Pamelor)

Common side effects caused by these medicines include dry mouth, blurred vision, constipation, difficulty urinating, worsening of glaucoma, impaired thinking, and tiredness. These antidepressants can also affect a person's blood pressure and heart rate. Tricyclic antidepressant medications can have drug interactions. You should consult with your doctor or pharmacist prior to mixing them with other medications.

- *Serotonin and norepinephrine reuptake inhibitors* (SNRIs):
    - venlafaxine (brand name: Effexor)
    - duloxetine (brand name: Cymbalta)

Some common side effects caused by these medicines include nausea and loss of appetite, anxiety and nervousness, headaches, insomnia, and tiredness. Dry mouth, constipation, weight loss, sexual problems, increased heart rate, and increased cholesterol levels can also occur.

- *Norepinephrine and dopamine reuptake inhibitors* (NDRIs):
    - bupropion (brand name: Wellbutrin)

Some of the common side effects in people taking NDRIs include agitation, nausea, headaches, loss of appetite, and insomnia. It can also cause increased blood pressure in some people.

- *Monamine oxidase inhibitors* (MAOIs):
    - isocarboxazid (brand name: Marplan)
    - phenelzine (brand name: Nardil)
    - tranlcypromine (brand name: Parnate)

MAOIs are used less commonly than the other antidepressants. They can have serious side effects, including weakness, dizziness, headaches, and trembling. Taking an MAOI antidepressant while you're aking another antidepressant or certain over-the-counter medicines for colds and flu can cause a dangerous reaction. MAOIs are very effective but have potentially life-threatening drug interactions and food interactions. If you are taking a MAOI drug, it is important that you consult with your doctor before you take any other medicines. Your doctor will also tell you which foods to avoid mixing with your medicine.

Antianxiety Medications

Antianxiety medications include the benzodiazepines, which can relieve symptoms within a short time. They have relatively few side effects: drowsiness and loss of coordination are most common; fatigue and mental slowing or confusion can also occur. These effects make it dangerous for people taking benzodiazepines to drive or operate some machinery. Commonly used benzodiazepines include clonazepam (*Klonopin*), alprazolam (*Xanax*), diazepam (*Valium*), and lorazepam (*Ativan*). A withdrawal reaction may occur if the treatment is stopped abruptly. Symptoms may include anxiety, shakiness, headache, dizziness, sleeplessness, loss of appetite, or, in extreme cases, seizures.

Exercise Therapy

Exercise is not only good for your health, it also can help you reduce depression. A recent study looked at exercise alone in treating mild to moderate depression. The researchers studied adults aged 20 to 45, finding that depressive symptoms were reduced almost 50 percent in individuals who participated in 30-minute aerobic exercise sessions three to five times a week.[30]

Relaxation Techniques

Relaxation techniques help individuals develop the ability to more effectively cope with the stresses that contribute to anxiety, as well as with some of the physical symptoms of anxiety. The techniques taught include breathing retraining and exercise.

The Role of Sleep

Insomnia refers to both the inability to fall asleep and a broken and restless sleep with early waking. Getting enough sleep is essential to having a healthy body, mind, and spirit. Sleep restores our bodies—it's when many important body functions occur, including tissue regeneration, muscle building, fat metabolism, blood sugar and insulin regulation, and time for conscious and unconscious mind communication. A baby needs 14 to 15 hours of sleep per day, and an adult needs 7 to 9 hours.

Effects of Chronic Sleep Deprivation

- Premature aging
- Obesity, diabetes (type 2) by increasing blood sugar
- Cortisol secretion

How to Get a Good Night's Sleep

- Regulate your body clock.
- Create a conductive sleep environment.
- Don't have caffeine, nicotine, or spicy food at night.
- Finish eating at least two hours before sleep.
- Limit computer and TV use before bed—soothing music and calm books are better choices.
- Meditation, visualization, and yoga can help with relaxation.
- Write in a journal.

Keep a Gratitude Journal

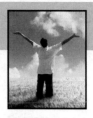

A gratitude journal is a way to consciously call attention to the things for which we are thankful each day. By focusing on gratitude, we become aware of those things and thus create a shift in our thinking to the positive. When you continuously express things you are grateful for, it trains your brain to begin focusing on things you like about your life instead of the things you don't. Many times depression stems from a routine of negative thoughts, so a gratitude journal re-programs your mind to think more positively. Begin looking every day for the positive in all things. View obstacles as *opportunities to appreciate.* The most powerful gratitude entries are ones where you **write down positive things about your negative situation**.

- Write a few things you're grateful for. Review the day and include anything, however small or great, that was a source of gratitude that day. Make the list personal. For example, say you're sad because you are overweight. Sure, you may write down you are happy to have a home, family, car, etc. in your journal, but it still may not help you feel better about your weight. That's when it's important to write down gratitude statements about your weight, which is what's *REALLY* bothering you, right? For example, you could say . . .

  1) *I am overweight but I love myself enough to want to eat healthier and change my body. And for that I'm grateful.*
  2) *I walked today and even though I was tired, I know it was good for me.*

Day 1

_____

_____

_____

_____

_____

Day 2

_____

_____

_____

_____

Day 3

_____

_____

_____

_____

Day 4

_____

_____

_____

_____

Day 5

_____

_____

_____

_____

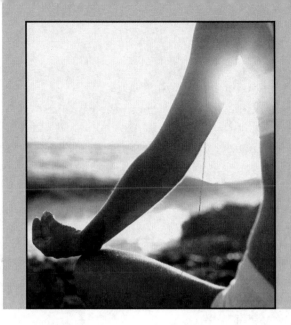

Chapter 3

Stress

Are You Under Stress?

I am physically tired.	Yes	No
I am emotionally tired.	Yes	No
I have headaches.	Yes	No
I have an upset stomach.	Yes	No
I have trouble sleeping.	Yes	No
I am irritable.	Yes	No
I am too tense.	Yes	No
I am angry.	Yes	No
I get into verbal/physical fights.	Yes	No
I have a hard time concentrating.	Yes	No
I am nervous.	Yes	No
I am worried.	Yes	No

Three or more "yes" answers can indicate stress.

What Do You Know About Stress?

True or False

1. Anxiety and stress are the same thing.
2. High stress levels and chronic stress can contribute to heart disease, high blood pressure and strokes, and can depress the immune system.
3. It is impossible to treat stress without seeking professional help.
4. Good stress helps keep us alert, motivates us to face challenges and drives us to solve problems.
5. Any challenge, whether a physical or a psychological one, is a source of stress, and challenging situations should be avoided in order to avoid stress.
6. Smoking a cigarette helps to relieve stress.

7. Drinking coffee reduces stress.

8. Exercise helps to build the body but it depletes the body of energy, causing stress.

9. Studies have indicated that people who "vent" their emotions by talking about their problems, writing about their problems, etc., are less likely to experience physical and psychological illness.

10. Stress management includes getting enough sleep, drinking enough water, eating healthy foods, getting enough exercise, and learning how to say "NO!".

Definition of Stress

To your body, *stress* is synonymous with change. Stress is the emotional and physical symptoms that individuals experience as the result of change. Stress may be considered as any physical, chemical, or emotional factor that causes bodily or mental tension and that may be a factor in disease causation. The majority of visits to physicians are because of stress-related complaints.

Stress can be positive or negative (eustress vs. distress). A mild degree of stress and tension can sometimes be beneficial.

Symptoms of Stress

- Rapid heart rate
- Headaches, backaches
- Muscular aches
- Sweating
- Tics
- Insomnia
- Fatigue
- High blood pressure
- Impotence and other sexual problems
- Dizziness
- Depression, anxiety
- Irritation, anger, hostility
- Fear, panic attacks
- Poor concentration
- More infections, illnesses

Types of Stress

- Emotional _____
- Physical _____
- Environmental _____

Episodes of Stress

- Acute _____
- Episodic _____
- Chronic _____

What Happens to Our Bodies Under Stress?

- *Brain*—headaches, anxiety, depression, insomnia, memory loss
- *Digestive system*—slows down; mouth ulcers or cold sores; upset stomach
- *Heart*—Increased heart rate, increased blood pressure
- *Skin*—breakouts, rashes, itching, eczema
- *Muscle*—tension, tics
- *Reproductive system*—menstrual disorders, infertility in females; impotence, premature ejaculation in males.

Stress and the Immune System

- Powerful chemicals triggered by stress suppress the immune system, making the body more susceptible to illness.
- Stress interferes with the body's ability to heal.
- Increased adrenaline production causes the body to increase metabolism of proteins, fats, and carbohydrates to quickly produce energy for the body to use.
- The pituitary gland increases production of andrenocorticotropic hormone (ACTH), which in turn stimulates the release of cortisone and cortisol hormones. These hormonal releases may inhibit the functioning of disease-fighting white blood cells and suppress the immune system's response.

Health Disorders Associated with Chronic Stress

- Coronary heart disease
- Hypertension
- Diabetes
- Progression of breast cancer
- Ulcers
- Eating disorders
- Asthma
- Depression
- Migraines
- Sleep disorders
- Chronic fatigue
- Physical aches, pains

Selye's Model—General Adaptation Syndrome

Stressor = Alarm → Resistance → Exhaustion

Our bodies try to keep in balance (homeostasis), but stress may upset that balance. Hans Selye explained stress through GAS (general adaptation syndrome), a way that the body tries to keep in balance.

A stressor is anything that affects you emotionally or physically.

Examples of Stressors

- School
- Work
- Parents
- Relationships
- Road rage
- Illness and disability
- Death of a loved one
- Discrimination
- Violence
- War
- Other

The *alarm stage* is when your body is preparing to defend itself against the stressor. Your body will go into "fight or flight" response by releasing hormones such as adrenaline and insulin to allow you to flee or attack. Heart rate and blood pressure will be elevated. In ancient times, a stressor such as being chased by a tiger would be beneficial by allowing the release of adrenaline hormones to allow for running away or killing the tiger.

The *resistance stage* allows arousal to be elevated while the body is trying to defend itself against the stressor.

The *exhaustion stage* occurs when resources are limited or depleted and the ability to resist the stressor is impaired. This stage leads to increased vulnerability of health problems and an impaired immune system.

Personality Types and Stress

- *Type A*—aggressive, hard-driven, impatient; high levels of distress. Prone to stress-related diseases such as ulcers, heart disease, hypertension, and certain cancers.
- *Type B*—easygoing, laid-back, patient; low levels of distress.
- *Type C*—passive, apologetic, overly sensitive; moderate levels of distress. Prone to stress-related mental disorders.
- *Type D*—tendency towards negativity; may experience a lot of stress, anger, worry, hostility, tension, and other negative and distressing emotions. Prone to depression, heart disease, hypertension.

Stress May Trigger Anger

Researchers believe that prolonged stress and anger, result in the breakdown of the cardiovascular system. It can also increase your risk for developing **mental health concerns** such as:

- Depression
- Eating disorders
- Drug, alcohol or other addictions
- Suicidal thoughts
- Relationship problems

You might be holding in anger and not even be aware of it. Do you find yourself flying off the handle on a regular basis or having road rage or screaming or exploding at the littlest things that aggravate you?

Anger is caused by an irrational perception of reality and a low frustration point. Angry people almost never admit responsibility—they blame something or someone else for their anger. When you are

46

in the angry "rage"—its hard to think clearly because your emotions take control of your actions. The fight or flight response takes over and increases blood pressure and heart rate and releases adrenaline into your bloodstream, which tells your body to either defend yourself, or attack someone/something.

How to Control Your Anger

- Breathe deeply, from your diaphragm.
- Slowly repeat a calming word or phrase such as "relax" or "calm."
- Use imagery; visualize a relaxing experience.
- Exercise or yoga to release the adrenaline.
- Take a "time out"—leave the scene and cool off.
- Talk with a psychologist to improve your problem-solving skills.

How to Deal With an Angry Person

1. Become an impartial observer—act as if you were watching someone else.
2. Stay calm—do not add fuel to the fire.
3. Refuse to engage.
4. Defuse them by ignoring them, looking away, or starting another conversation with a totally different topic, or find something you can agree with or praise them.
5. Walk away if the person is getting out of control.
6. Practice your deep breathing.

How to Change Your Personality to Become More Stress-Resilient

- Build greater social support networks.
- Participate in and contribute to your community in productive ways.
- Set clear boundaries and expectations for yourself.
- Develop decision-making skills.
- Practice effective communication techniques.
- Learn conflict management techniques.
- Do not try to control the outcome of every situation.

Hardiness—health authorities have now identified the concept of hardiness as a characteristic that has helped people negate self-imposed stress.

One researcher in the stress hardiness field is the clinical psychologist at City University, New York, Susan Kobasa, PhD. In the late 1970s she carried out a study on a group of executives who were under a lot of stress while their company, the Bell Telephone Company, was undergoing radical restructuring. On completion of the study, when the data was analyzed, she found that certain personality traits protected some of the executives and managers from the health ravages of stress.

These stress-hardy personality traits included:

1. **Commitment**—having a purpose to life and involvement in family, work, community, social friends, religious faith, ourselves, etc., giving us a meaning to our lives.
2. **Control**—studies have shown that how much control we perceive we have over any stressor will influence how difficult the stressor will be for us to cope with.
3. **Challenge**—how we perceive the events that occur in our lives; seeing our difficulties as a challenge rather than as a threat, and accepting that the only thing in life that is constant, is change.

> You can't always influence what others may say or do to you
> but you can influence how you react and respond to it.
>
> *(Unknown)*

Definitions

Hormone: A chemical substance released into the body by the endocrine glands such as the thyroid, adrenal, or ovaries. The substance travels through the bloodstream and sets in motion various body functions. For example, prolactin, which is produced in the pituitary gland, begins and sustains the production of breastmilk after childbirth.[31]

Neurotransmitters: Specialized chemical messengers (e.g., acetylcholine, dopamine, norepinephrine, serotonin) that send messages from one nerve cell to another. Most neurotransmitters play different roles throughout the body, many of which are not yet known.[32]

Neurotransmitters are molecules that regulate brain function. They are chemicals that relay messages from nerve to nerve both within the brain and outside the brain. They also relay messages from nerve to muscle, lungs, and intestinal tracts. They can accentuate *emotion, thought processes, joy, elation*, and also *fear, anxiety, insomnia*, and the terrible urge to *overindulge* in food, alcohol, drugs, and so on. In short, neurotransmitters are used all over the body to transmit information and signals. They are manufactured and used by neurons (nerve cells) and are released into the synaptic clefts between the neurons.

Currently, over 50 neurotransmitters have been identified, and it is estimated that around 100 neurotransmitters exist in the biological systems.

Stress Hormones/Neurotransmitters

Epinephrine, also known as *adrenaline*, the major stress neurotransmitter, is related to blood pressure and heart rate. Adrenaline prepares the body for "fright, fight, or flight" responses and has many effects, including:

- Action of heart increased
- Rate and depth of breathing increased
- Metabolic rate increased
- Force of muscular contraction improves
- Onset of muscular fatigue delayed

Norepinephrine, also known as *noradrenaline*, is a second stress neurotransmitter. High levels of this hormone are seen in states of anxiety and insomnia. It is released in response to perceived threat. The effects of the hormone noradrenaline are similar to the effects of adrenaline, the other hormone secreted by the adrenal medulla.

The actions of noradrenaline include:

- Constriction of small blood vessels leading to increase in blood pressure
- Increased blood flow through the coronary arteries and slowing of heart rate
- Increase in rate and depth of breathing

Increased amounts of both adrenaline and noradrenaline are secreted when the body is under stress.

48

Cortisol is secreted in times of stress. Cortisol stimulates fat and carbohydrate metabolism for fast energy, and stimulates insulin release and maintenance of blood sugar levels. The end result of these actions is *an increase in appetite*, especially cravings for sugared foods. Cortisol increases abdominal obesity. Cortisol secretion is highest in people who sleep less than six hours per night.

Major "Happy" Neurotransmitters

- *Endorphins* (opioids): Provides mood-elevating, enhancing, and euphoric effects. The more endorphins present, the happier you are! Endorphins are like natural painkillers—your body's natural heroin.

- *Dopamine:* Runs your body's pleasure center. Creates feelings of bliss and pleasure, euphoria, and focus. Also leads to appetite control and controlled motor movements. Modulates the effect of the excitatory hormones, and is necessary for states of relaxation and mental alertness.

- *Serotonin:* Manufactured from tryptophan. It is found all over the body and is necessary to modulate the levels of the stress hormones. Promotes and improves sleep, improves self-esteem, relieves depression, diminishes craving, and prevents agitated depression and worrying. Converts to melatonin and then back to serotonin. Regulates your body clock. First to fail under stress.

- *Melatonin:* "Rest and recuperation" and "antiaging" hormone. Regulates body clock.

- *Acetylcholine:* Affects alertness, memory, and sexual performance; stimulates appetite control, and release of growth hormone.

- *Phenylethylamine (PEA):* Provides feelings of bliss, feelings of infatuation (high levels are found in chocolate).

- *Oxytocin:* Stimulated by dopamine. Promotes sexual arousal, feelings of emotional attachment, and desire to cuddle.

- *GABA (gamma amino butyric acid):* Found throughout central nervous system, produces antistress, antianxiety, antipanic, and antipain effects. Allows individual to feel calm, maintain control, and focus.

Neurotransmitters control

- Nicotine craving
- Premenstrual syndrome (PMS)
- Irritable bowel
- Caffeine craving
- ADHD
- Anorexia and bulimia
- Migraine headache
- Panic attacks
- Alcohol craving
- Leg cramps
- Constipation
- Carbohydrate cravings
- OCD
- Aggression
- Impulsivity

How Stress Affects Neurotransmitters

The brain uses feel-good transmitters called endorphins when managing daily stress. When the brain requires larger amounts of endorphins to handle increased stress, the ratio of many of the other transmitters, one to another, becomes upset, creating a chemical imbalance. We begin to feel stress more acutely—a sense of urgency and anxiety creates even more stress. As long as the brain has a balanced amount of happy and sad messengers, everything runs smoothly and we are in homeostasis.

It is imperative that all of the major neurotransmitters be present daily and in sufficient amounts in order for the brain to be chemically balanced. When insufficient amounts of one or more of these neurotransmitters exists, it upsets the ratio and symptoms are experienced.

Depleted supplies of feel-good transmitters means it will be impossible for you to feel happy, upbeat, motivated, or on track. You will feel just the opposite: a decrease in energy and interest, feelings of worthlessness, and a pervasive sense of helplessness to control the course of your life.

Certain transmitters, when depleted, may cause you to be easily agitated or angered, experience mild to severe anxiety, and have sleep problems. You may feel more psychological and physical pain. These are all possible symptoms of neurotransmitter deficiencies.

Main Causes of Neurotransmitter Deficiencies

- *Genetics:* A person's genetic makeup is responsible for low, high, or balanced levels of transmitters from birth.
- *Stress:* Stress depletes neurotransmitters! Any type of stress (lack of sleep, everyday mental and emotional battles, or poor health) will deplete feel-good transmitters. This results in a reduction of transmitters needed for sleep, as well as a reduction in pain-blocking transmitters.
- *Diet:* The specific amino acids that our brains manufacture transmitters from are frequently not supplied by our modern diet or in the way our brain best utilizes them. Nutrient-depleted soils, fruits and vegetables not allowed to fully ripen on the vine, and overprocessing of foods have all combined over the last century to rob our diets of many life-giving nutrients. Experts in the field of brain nutrition all agree that it is very difficult to get the necessary supply of the specific amino acids from our American diet that our brain needs to create enough of the neurotransmitters that keep us feeling balanced and happy.

How to Treat Neurotransmitter Imbalance

If we treat a neurotransmitter imbalance with pharmaceutical medication (i.e., the serotonin reuptake inhibitors like Prozac, Celexa, Paxil, and Zoloft), we tend to impose an artificial and imbalanced level of a specific neurotransmitter.

These drugs will increase the amount of serotonin at the synaptic cleft, causing the body to *think* that serotonin levels are higher. Most people will feel better temporarily. When serotonin stores fall below a certain level, the medication "stops working" and a different medication must be used. However, they do *not increase the total body stores of serotonin,* and therefore are not the best permanent solution.

Alternatives to Medication

1. Increase dietary intake of tryptophan. American diets tend to be high in carbohydrate and low in protein. Foods high in tryptophan are mostly high-protein foods:
   - Cottage cheese—450 mg per cup
   - Fish and other seafood—800–1,300 mg per pound
   - Meats—1,000–1,300 mg per pound
   - Poultry—600–1,200 mg per pound
   - Peanuts, roasted with skin—800 mg per cup

- Sesame seeds—700 mg per cup
- Dry, whole lentils—450 mg/cup

2. Increase amount of exercise. Exercise leads to more efficient use of insulin, thus reducing insulin resistance and decreasing the amount of food that is stored as fat. When the cells process nutrients better, they make neurotransmitters better. Exercise releases endorphins, which are natural mood elevators.

3. Reduce our intake of caffeine. Caffeine makes the body think is it under stress, which raises the cortisol level, raises the insulin level, and causes carbohydrates to be deposited as fat.

Functions of Endorphins

Endorphins, chemicals produced in the brain in response to a variety of stimuli, may be nature's cure for high levels of stress.

Endorphins are among the brain chemicals known as neurotransmitters, which, as noted, function in the transmission of signals within the nervous system. At least 20 types of endorphins have been demonstrated in humans, and they may be located in the pituitary gland, other parts of the brain, or distributed throughout the nervous system.

Stress and pain are the two most common factors leading to the release of endorphins. Endorphins interact with the opiate receptors in the brain to reduce our perception of pain, having a similar action to drugs such as morphine and codeine. Unlike drugs, however, activation of the opiate receptors by the body's endorphins does not lead to addiction or dependence.

Results of Endorphin Secretion

- Decreased feelings of pain
- Feelings of euphoria
- Modulation of appetite
- Release of sex hormones
- Enhancement of the immune response

Stress and Digestion

Stress contributes to ulcers and ailing digestion.

- Good nutrition can help.
- Complex carbohydrates increase levels of serotonin.
- Stay hydrated with water to compensate for fluid lost during sweating under stress and stress-induced dry mouth.
- Eat frequent, small meals to maintain normal blood sugar, prevent fatigue and irritability, and prevent slow metabolism.
- Avoid overeating, which can increase stress.
- Limit consumption of sugar, caffeine, nicotine, and alcohol.

Vitamin and Mineral Deficiencies

Chronic stress can deplete several vitamins necessary for energy metabolism, as well as those necessary for the stress response itself. The stress response activates several hormones responsible for mobilizing and metabolizing fats and carbohydrates for energy production. The breakdown of fats and carbohydrates requires vitamins, specifically the B vitamins and vitamin C. An inadequate supply of these may affect mental alertness, promote depression, and lead to insomnia. Stress is also associated with the depletion of calcium and the inability of bones to absorb it properly.

"Pick-Me-Ups" and Stress

When people are stressed, they use *pick-me-ups* or *put-me-downs* to combat the stressor. Several substances tend to either mimic or induce the stress response, or decrease the efficiency of the body's metabolic pathways, thus setting the stage for more pronounced physiological reactions to stress. The biggest mistake people make in handling stress is using pick-me-ups to boost happy messengers, which has the effect of riding a wild roller coaster.

Sugar: Excess sugar tends to deplete vitamin stores, especially the B vitamins that are crucial for optimal function of the central nervous system. Depletion of B vitamins may result in fatigue, anxiety, and irritability. In addition, excess simple sugars can cause major fluctuations in blood glucose levels, resulting in pronounced fatigue, headaches, and irritability.

Simple Sugars

- Glucose (honey)
- Lactose (milk)
- Fructose (fruit)
- Sucrose (cane)

Fats: You've likely heard all the bad news about how fat creates artery-clogging cholesterol and weight gain. But a high-fat diet also leaves you feeling lethargic and just not feeling as well as you would on a diet high in complex carbohydrates.

Caffeine: Caffeine stimulates the release of several stress hormones, resulting in a state of hyper-alertness, and makes a person more likely to interpret events as stressful.

Alcohol: Increases short-term energy, but then blood sugar dips. Diminishes pain, but can lead to aggression and depression.

Salt: High sodium acts to increase water retention, and as water volume increases, blood pressure increases. Habitual high sodium intake may contribute to hypertension.

Tobacco: Powerful toxin; destroys trachea, bronchi, and lung function. Damages arteries, causing insufficient blood supply to the brain, heart, and organs. Carcinogenic. Increases dopamine but levels fall shortly, requiring more nicotine.

Drugs: Increases release of dopamine (pleasure center), shutting off brain's natural supply.

Your own adrenaline: Allows body to prepare for fight or flight. For example, a workaholic who is overstressed → works longer hours → feeds off his own adrenaline.

Put-Me-Downs

▨ *"Doctor, can you give me something to calm me down?"*

Medications that temporarily force the body into sleeping, producing a tranquilizing effect, are referred to as *put-me-downs*. These medications produce addiction and severe withdrawal symptoms.

- Valium, Xanax, Ativan
- Barbiturates

52

Stress Interventions

1. Do a minimum of 30 minutes of aerobic exercise daily, or take a walk.
2. Make your body clock regular.
3. Eat five small, balanced meals per day.
4. Avoid caffeine, drugs, and tobacco.
5. Reduce intake of refined sugars and alcohol.
6. Sleep about eight hours nightly.
7. Spend time each day with relaxation techniques—imagery, daydreaming, prayer, or meditation.
8. Take a warm bath or shower.
9. Listen to music; watch a comedy.
10. Postpone making changes in your life.
11. Hug someone, hold hands, or stroke a pet.
12. Pray.

Techniques to Handle Stress

1. *Deep breathing:* Inhale through your nose slowly, counting silently to five, and then exhale through your mouth slowly, counting silently to five.
2. *Positive affirmations:* Talk in a positive manner to yourself; turn your negative comments into positive ones: "*I will pass the test.*"
3. *Stretching:* Stretch the area where tension has built up, holding for 30 seconds; relax and repeat three to five times.
4. *Progressive muscle relaxation:* Tense a muscle and hold it for a silent, slow count of 5–10 seconds, then release the muscle for a silent, slow count 5–10 seconds.
5. *Visualization:* Find a quiet space, get comfortable, close your eyes, and try to imagine yourself in a calm, enjoyable, relaxing setting. Think about the details of your tranquil setting. Who is with you? How is the weather? What does it smell like?
6. *Meditation:* Find a quiet space, get comfortable, close your eyes, and begin breathing deeply. Focus on one image or thought. Try this for 5–10 minutes every day.
7. *Yoga:* Used since ancient times to invigorate the body and calm the mind.
8. *Massage:* Research indicates that human touch is vital for well-being.
9. *Pets:* Animals decrease stress levels through touch, companionship.
10. *Talk to someone:* A friend, parent, teacher, or a college counselor.

Free and confidential counseling:
Queensborough College Counseling Center—Library Room 428,
718-631-6370 or www.qcc.cuny.edu/counseling

How to Conquer Test Anxiety[33]

- Prepare well in advance—rehearsal and repetition.
- Get a good night's sleep—eight hours.
- Eat a nutritious meal to boost your brain's energy.

- Have a positive attitude—go in with a positive attitude, reminding yourself that you are well prepared.
- If you stumble on a question, don't linger on it. Go on to the next question.
- Ask for clarification if you don't understand the question.
- Don't pay attention to the people around you—stay focused on the test and don't get distracted.
- Take deep breaths, bringing more oxygen to the brain.
- Pace yourself—be aware of the time.

How to Manage Your Time

- Rank tasks in order of importance.
- Schedule a time frame for each task.
- List your deadlines on a calendar or daily planner.
- Delegate and ask for help with some tasks.
- Say no if demands are unreasonable.
- Schedule personal time in your daily planner for exercise, a hobby, or meditation, and stick to that schedule.
- Watch less television (1 hour per day).

Mindful Meditation

Meditation is the practice of seeing clearly, the art of moment-to-moment awareness, a nonjudgmental quality of mind that is aware of what is happening in and around oneself in the *present moment*.[34]

How to Mindfully Meditate

- Begin by sitting in a chair or on a cushion on the floor, with your back straight. Relax into your sitting posture with a few deep breaths. Allow the body and mind to become utterly relaxed while remaining very alert and attentive to the present moment. Feel the areas of your body that are tense and the areas that are relaxing. Just let the body follow its own natural law. Do not try to force or fix anything.
- Let your mind be soft, and allow a spacious awareness to wash gently through your body. Simply feel the sensations of sitting, sidestepping with your mind the tendency to see your body—to interpret, define, or think about it. Just let such thoughts and images come and go without being bothered by them, and attune to the bare sensations of sitting.
- Feel your body with an awareness that arises from within your body, not from your head. Awareness of the body anchors your attention in the present moment. Gently sweep your awareness through your body, feeling the sensations with no agenda, no goal. Allow your body to anchor awareness in the present moment by just staying mindful of these sensations.
- After some time, shift your awareness to the field of sound vibrations. Awareness of sounds creates openness, spaciousness, and receptivity in the mind. Be aware of both the pure sound vibration as well as the space or silence between the sounds. As with body sensations, incline your awareness away from the definition of the sound, or thoughts about the sound, and simply attune to the sound just as it is.
- After some minutes of awareness of body and sounds, bring your attention to your natural breathing process. Locate the area where the breath is most clear and let awareness lightly rest there.

For some it is the sensation of the rising and falling of the abdomen. For others it may be the sensations experienced at the nostrils with inhalation and exhalation.

- You can use very soft mental labels to guide and sustain attention to the breath, such as "rising/falling" for the abdomen and "in/out" for the nostrils. Let the breath breathe itself without control, direction, or force. Feel each breath from within the breath, not from the head. Feel the full breath cycle from the beginning through the middle to the end.

- The awareness is a combination of light, open spaciousness and receptivity, like listening, and alert, attentive presence, touching the actual texture, shape, and form of sensations.

- Let go of everything else, or let it be in the background. Just let the breathing breathe itself. Rest in a sense of utter relaxation, in that mindful feeling, with the sensations of the breath.

- As soon as you notice the mind wandering off, lost in thought, be aware of that with nonjudging awareness; gently connect it again to your anchor. Just feel from within the stream of sensations.

- Toward the end of your sitting, not striving or anticipating, not pouncing on sensations in the present, not bending back to what was just missed or reflecting on what just happened, keep inclining to the totality of the present moment. Keep anchoring easily, deeply, and restfully. Just one breath at a time.

- Mindfulness of breath begins to collect and concentrate the mind so that the initial distractions of thoughts, emotions, sensations, and sounds soon become objects of awareness themselves. Insight is gained into the true nature of the body and mind.

- As concentration grows, mindfulness opens to the entire "flow" of body/mind experience through all the sense doors—sights, sounds, smells, tastes, touch, and mental/emotive.[35]

Progressive Muscle Relaxation

One of the most simple and easily learned techniques for relaxation is progressive muscle relaxation (PMR), a widely used procedure that was originally developed by Jacobson in 1939.[36] The PMR procedure teaches you to relax your muscles through a two-step process. First, you deliberately apply tension to certain muscle groups, and then you stop the tension and turn your attention to noticing how the muscles relax as the tension flows away. Before practicing PMR, you should consult with your physician if you have a history of serious injuries, muscle spasms, or back problems, because the deliberate muscle tensing of the PMR procedure could exacerbate any of these preexisting conditions.

How to Get Started

Sit in a comfortable chair or bed. Get as comfortable as possible—no tight clothes, no shoes, don't cross your legs. Take a deep breath; let it out slowly. What you'll be doing is alternately tensing and relaxing specific groups of muscles. After tension, a muscle will be more relaxed than prior to the tensing. Concentrate on the feel of the muscles, specifically the contrast between tension and relaxation. In time, you will recognize tension in any specific muscle and be able to reduce that tension.

Don't tense muscles other than the specific group at each step. Don't hold your breath, grit your teeth, or squint! Breathe slowly and evenly and think only about the tension-relaxation contrast. Each tensing is for 10 seconds; each relaxing is for 10 or 15 seconds. Count "1,000, 2,000 . . ." until you have a feel for the time span. Note that each step is really two steps—one cycle of tension-relaxation for each set of opposing muscles.

Do the entire sequence once a day if you can, until you feel you are able to control your muscle tensions. Be careful: If you have problems with pulled muscles, broken bones, or any medical contraindication for physical activities, ***consult your doctor first.***

1. *Hands.* The fists are tensed; relaxed. The fingers are extended; relaxed.

2. *Biceps and triceps.* The biceps are tensed (make a muscle, but shake your hands to make sure not tensing them into a fist); relaxed (drop your arm to the chair—really drop them). The triceps are tensed (try to bend your arms the wrong way); relaxed (drop them).

3. *Shoulders.* Pull them back (careful with this one); relax them. Push the shoulders forward (hunch); relax.

4. *Neck* (lateral). With the shoulders straight and relaxed, the head is turned slowly to the right, as far as you can; relax. Turn to the left; relax.

5. *Neck* (forward). Dig your chin into your chest; *relax.* **(Bringing the head back is not recommended— you could break your neck).**

6. *Mouth.* The mouth is opened as far as possible; relaxed. The lips are brought together or pursed as tightly as possible; relaxed.

7. *Tongue* (extended and retracted). With mouth open, extend the tongue as far as possible; relax (let it sit in the bottom of your mouth). Bring it back in your throat as far as possible; relax.

8. *Tongue* (roof and floor). Dig your tongue into the roof of your mouth; relax. Dig it into the bottom of your mouth; relax.

9. *Eyes.* Open them as wide as possible (furrow your brow); relax. Close your eyes tightly (squint); relax. Make sure you completely relax the eyes, forehead, and nose after each of the tensings.

10. *Breathing.* Take as deep a breath as possible—and then take a little more; let it out and breathe normally for 15 seconds. Let all the breath in your lungs out—and then a little more; inhale and breathe normally for 15 seconds.

11. *Back.* With shoulders resting on the back of the chair, push your body forward so that your back is arched; relax. Be very careful with this one, or don't do it at all.

12. *Buttocks.* Tense the buttocks tightly and raise pelvis slightly off chair; relax. Dig buttocks into chair; relax.

13. *Thighs.* Extend legs and raise them about 6″ off the floor or the footrest—but don't tense the stomach—relax. Dig your feet (heels) into the floor or footrest; relax.

14. *Stomach.* Pull in the stomach as far as possible; relax completely. Push out the stomach or tense it as if you were preparing for a punch in the gut; relax.

15. *Calves and feet.* Point the toes (without raising the legs); relax. Point the feet up as far as possible (beware of cramps—if you get them or feel them coming on, shake them loose); relax.

16. *Toes.* With legs relaxed, dig your toes into the floor; relax. Bend the toes up as far as possible; relax.

Now just relax for a while. As your days of practice progress, you may wish to skip the body areas that do not appear to be a problem for you. After you've become an expert on your tension areas (after a few weeks), you can concern yourself only with those. These exercises will not eliminate tension, but when it arises, you will know it immediately, and you will be able to "tense-relax" it away or even simply wish it away.[37]

Stress Awareness Log

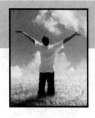

A daily record of stressors can serve as a valuable tool in learning to cope with stress. For at least 3 days, keep a log of all the situations that were stressful to you. What physical or mental symptoms did you exhibit? How did you deal with the stressor—was that an effective strategy or what else should you have done?

Date	Stressor	Symptoms	How did I deal—effective or not?

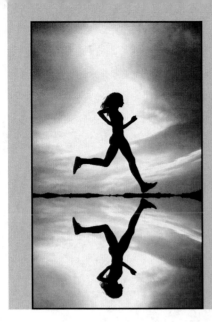

Chapter 4
Fitness

Physical fitness is not only one of the most important keys to a healthy body, it is the basis of dynamic and creative intellectual activity.
—*John. F. Kennedy*

Regular exercise has many positive benefits—from decreased health risk to weight management to stress reduction. Reflect on some ways that exercise can impact your life.

_____

_____

_____

_____

_____

_____

_____

Why You Should Exercise Regularly?

1. Exercise helps to elevate your mood.
2. Exercise can help you achieve and maintain a healthy weight.
3. Regular exercise will help you sleep better at night.
4. Exercise strengthens your heart and lungs.
5. Being physically active can improve your sex life.
6. Exercise combats chronic diseases.
7. Exercise boosts your energy level.

8. Exercise boosts brain power.
9. Exercise increases your metabolism.
10. Exercise increases your immune system.
11. Exercise increases life expectancy and lowers mortality.

Mental Health Benefits of Physical Activity

- Reduced anxiety
- Reduced depression
- Increased positive self-esteem
- Better sleep quality

Exercise and Endorphins

Many fitness enthusiasts experience something called a "runner's high." You actually don't have to run a marathon to experience this high—moderate exercise releases endorphins which act as powerful hormone-like substances produced in the brain that function as the body's own natural painkillers. During exercise, there is a release of endorphins in the body that are capable of producing feelings of euphoria and a general state of well-being. The feelings produced can be so powerful that they can actually mask pain.

Sedentary Death Syndrome[38]

- Every year in the United States, approximately 300,000 deaths occur due to physical inactivity.
- In the next decade, an expected 2.5 million premature deaths will occur.
- This results in billions of dollars in health-care costs each year.

Characteristics of Sedentary People

- Higher risk of heart attacks
- Higher risk of certain cancers
- Higher risk of hypertension
- Higher risk of osteoporosis
- Greater number of sick days
- Higher stress
- Greater depression and anxiety
- Greater appetite

Inactivity Epidemic[39]

- One in four Americans report no physical activity
- City dwellers versus country folks
- Female versus males
- Higher education versus lower education
- Higher income versus lower income

Children and Inactivity

- Less active
- Higher rates of obesity
- Decreased physical education classes
- Increased diabetes, hypertension, risk of heart disease
- Lower academic performance

College Students

Do you exercise? Why or why not?

_____

_____

_____

_____

_____

List some reasons why college students do not exercise.

_____

_____

_____

_____

_____

How can we motivate college students to exercise?

_____

_____

_____

_____

_____

Why College Students Exercise—or Don't[40]

Top Exercise Benefits

- Exercise increases my level of physical fitness.
- Exercise improves the way my body looks.
- My muscle tone is improved with exercise.
- Exercise gives me a sense of personal accomplishment.
- Exercise increases my muscle strength.

Top Exercise Barriers

- Exercise tires me.
- Exercise is hard work for me.
- I am fatigued by exercise.
- Exercising takes too much time.
- My family members do not encourage me to exercise.
- No money to join a gym.

Barrier Busters

- Education
- Planning on calendar in ink
- Keeping sneakers in car
- Social support
- Park a few blocks away
- Take stairs
- Take 10-minute walks several times a day
- Hop off the bus/train early and walk
- Turn household chores into calorie burners
- Sign up for a fitness class
- Read schoolwork on stationary bike or stairmaster
- Rewards

Transtheoretical Model (Stages of Change)[41]

James Prochaska and Carlo Diclemente (1982) developed a model of change that is unique in many ways. The model conceptualizes change as entailing a number of stages, which all require alterations in attitude in order to progress. The model depicts change as a cycle as opposed to an all-or-nothing step. The authors contend that it is quite normal for people to require several trips through the stages to make lasting change. Thus, in this sense relapse is viewed as a normal part of the change process as opposed to a complete failure. This does not mean that relapse is desirable or even invariably expected. It simply means that change is difficult, and it is unreasonable to expect everyone to be able to modify a habit perfectly without any slips. The reason the cycle model is so attractive is that it views change as flexible to individual needs. Some people make lasting change quite rapidly; others require a few times through the stages.[42]

Are You Ready to Become More Active?

Precontemplation: No intention to take action within the next six months.

Contemplation: Intends to take action within the next six months.

Preparation: Intends to take action within the next 30 days and has taken some behavioral steps in this direction.

Action: Has changed overt behavior for less than six months.

Maintenance: Has changed overt behavior for more than six months.

Termination: Overt behavior will never return; complete confidence in ability to cope without relapse.

Process of change: Any activity that you initiate to help soothe your thinking, feeling, or behavior.

Nine Major Processes of Change

1. *Consciousness Raising*—Involves providing information regarding the nature and risk of unsafe behaviors and the value and drawbacks of the safer behavioral alternatives.

2. *Dramatic Relief*—Fosters the identification, experiencing, and expression of emotions related to the risk of the safer alternatives in order to work toward adaptive behavior.

3. *Environmental Control*—Allows the individual to reflect on the consequences of his or her behavior for other people. It can include reconsideration of perceptions of social norms and the opinions of people considered important.

4. *Self-Reevaluation*—Entails the reappraisal of one's problem and the kind of person one is able to be, given the problem.

5. *Commitment*—Encourages the person to consider his or her confidence in the ability to change and his or her commitment to doing so.

6. *Social Liberation*—Seeking to help others with similar situations.

7. *Helping Relationships*—Assist the person in a variety of ways, including providing emotional support, modeling a set of moral beliefs, and serving as a sounding board.

8. *Rewards*—Developing internal and external rewards and making them readily but contingently available to improve the probability of the new behavior occurring or continuing.

9. *Countering*—Weighing the pros and cons of the behavior change. The challenge is to tip the balance in favor of making positive changes.

Describe what stage of change you are currently in.

_____

_____

_____

_____

_____

_____

Definitions of Physical Fitness

Physical fitness: Ability to respond to routine physical demands with enough reserve energy to cope with a sudden change.

Aerobic: Oxygen taken into the body is greater than amount of oxygen used by the body.

Examples of aerobic activity:

- Walking
- Jogging/running
- Cycling
- Skiing
- Dancing
- Skating
- Swimming
- Rowing
- Stair climber

Which aerobic activity do you currently perform or would like to start for this semester?

_____

_____

_____

_____

_____

Cardiorespiratory endurance: The ability of the body's circulatory and respiratory systems to supply fuel during sustained physical activity.

Endorphins: Mood-elevating, pain-killing chemicals produced by the brain.

Healthy Benefits of Aerobic Exercise[43]

- Reduction in body weight
- Reduction in blood pressure
- Reduction of low-density lipoprotein (LDL) and total cholesterol
- Increase in high-density lipoprotein (HDL) cholesterol
- Increased insulin sensitivity
- Larger coronary arteries
- Increased heart size
- Increased pumping action
- Increases stamina
- Reduces number of sick days
- Decreases risk of cancer

- Decreases risk of diabetes
- Decreases arthritis symptoms

Anaerobic: High-intensity activity that does not require oxygen to produce the desired energy to carry out the activity. Systems that create energy for activities that last less than five minutes or have frequent rest periods.

Examples of anaerobic activity:

- Sprinting
- Weight lifting

Muscle strength: Force within muscles; measured by the absolute maximum weight you can lift, push, or press.

Muscle endurance: Repeated muscular effort; measured by counting how many times you lift, push, or press a given weight.

Flexibility: Range of motion around specific joints.

Body composition: Relative amounts of fat and lean tissue in body.

- *Body mass index (BMI)*—over 25 is overweight; over 30 is obesity.
- *Waist size*—men with waists larger than 40 inches and women with waists larger than 35 inches are at greatest risk of heart disease.
- *Waist-to-hip ratio (WHR)*—greater than 1 for men or 85 for women is associated with greater risk.
- *Skinfold fat measurement*—a caliper is used to measure the amount of skinfold. Ideal body fat percentages for men are from 7 to 24 percent and for women from 16 to 31 percent.
- *Bioelectrical impedence analysis (BIA)*—noninvasive method; electrical current applied to the body. Based on the theory that lean tissue, which contains large amounts of water and electrolytes, is a good electrical conductor. Fat is a poor conductor.
- *Hydrostatic (underwater) weighing*—gold standard; involves suspending a person attached to a scale in water. Calculated from the relationship of normal body weight to underwater weight.
- *Dual-energy x-ray absorptiometry (DXA)*—x-rays used to quantify the skeletal and soft tissue components of body mass.
- *The Bod Pod*—large fiberglass chamber uses the relationship between pressure and volume to derive body volume.

Check Your Health Status Before Starting an Exercise Program

The American Heart Association and the American College of Sports Medicine (ACSM) recommend that you see a doctor before exercising if:[44]

- you have a heart condition.
- you take medicine for your heart and/or blood pressure.
- you get pains in your chest, left side of your neck, or your left shoulder or arm when you exercise.
- your chest has been hurting for about a month.
- you tend to get dizzy, lose consciousness.
- mild exertion leaves you breathless.
- you are overweight or obese.
- you have diabetes.
- you are over 50 years for women and over 40 for men.

Essential Components of an Exercise Program (FITT)

- *Frequency*—number of sessions per day and week
- *Intensity*—relative physiological difficulty of exercise; risk higher with intensity
- *Type* of exercise based on goals
- *Time*—length of session; inversely related with intensity and compliance

How Much Exercise Is Enough?[45]

The ACSM and the U.S. Surgeon General recommend a minimum of 30 to 60 minutes of moderate activity most days of the week to reduce the risk of cardiovascular disease.

- Aerobics 3–5 times/week; 20–60 minutes; 60–85 percent intensity
- Strength 2–3 times/week; 8–12 repetitions; 2–3 sets per muscle group
- Flexibility 2–3 times/week; especially on the days of strength training

Phases of Exercise Session

1. Warm-up: 5–10 minutes
2. Stretching: 5–10 minutes
3. Workout
4. Cool-down: 5–10 minutes
5. Stretch: 5 minutes

Why Warm Up?

- Prepares your body for physical activity by gradually increasing muscle temperature and metabolism
- Increases blood flow and oxygen delivery to the muscles, protects tendons, and lengthens short, tight muscles
- Gives the body a chance to redirect blood to active muscles
- Gives the heart time to adapt to increased demands
- Stretches the major joints with range-of-motion movements

Why Cool Down?

- Light, gradual movements and stretching to end your physical activity constitute a cool-down.
- Cool-down helps to avoid the pooling of blood in the muscles and to remove metabolic end-products such as lactic acid and carbon dioxide.
- Cool-down reduces muscle soreness, cramps, and stiffness.
- Stretching at the end improves flexibility and prevents injury.

Long-Term Plan of an Exercise Program

1. Beginning (4–6 weeks)—Start slow and with low intensity.
2. Progression (16–20 weeks)—Gradually increase the duration and intensity.
3. Maintenance (lifelong)—Once you've reached the stage of exercising for an hour every day, vary your intensity and duration.

Principles of a Successful Workout

- *Overload*—Placing a greater-than-normal amount of stress on the body in order to make it function at a higher capacity, therefore increasing endurance and/or strength.
- *Specificity*—The type of physical changes you desire in your body relate directly to the type of exercise you choose.
- *Progression*—By gradually increasing the frequency, intensity, and duration of exercise, the body is able to gain improvement in strength and endurance.
- *Intensity*—
    1. *Sedentary* individuals should work toward performing a minimum of 30 minutes of daily moderate activity to decrease risk of cardiovascular disease.
    2. *Moderate* intensity—activities that use energy three to six times the resting metabolic rate (RMR) (40–60 percent max).
    3. *Vigorous*—activities more than six times the RMR (60 percent max).

Heart Rate

- Total number of times the heart contracts per minute; normal rate is 60–80 bpm.
- The quicker your heart recovers after exercise, the better your physical health.
- Use radial or carotid artery for measurement.
- Resting heart rate is most accurately measured upon awakening in the morning.

Estimate Your Maximum Heart Rate[46]

- Take 220 – age = _____ (this is your maximum); standard deviation for this equation is 10–12 beats per minute.
- Determine your lower-limit exercise heart rate by multiplying your maximum heart rate by 0.6 (60 percent intensity).
- Determine your upper-limit exercise rate heart by multiplying your maximum heart rate by 0.8 (80 percent intensity).

Your exercise heart rate range is between your upper and lower limits.

For most people, exercising at the lower end of the exercise heart rate range for a longer time is better than exercising at the higher end of the range for a shorter time. Exercising at the lower intensity will improve your overall fitness.

Medications for high blood pressure may affect your heart rate during exercise.

Target Heart Rate (Fat-Burning Zone)

220 – AGE = _____

_____ × .60 = _____ low end of target zone

_____ × .80 = _____ high end of target zone

- Use 60 to 85 percent of your heart rate (HR).
- For weight loss, use 60 to 70 percent of max HR.
- For aerobic conditioning, use 70 to 80 percent of HR.
- If you exercise at higher intensity, it can place a burden on the heart.
- If you don't exercise hard enough, weight loss is impeded.

Target Heart Rate Formula for Women

In a recent study from Northwestern University of nearly 5,500 healthy women, scientists discovered that a decades-old formula for calculating heart rate is largely inaccurate for women, resulting in a number that is too high.

The new formula is:

206 − (0.88 × age) = _____ estimated max heart rate.

The typical goal is to stay within 65 to 85 percent of the estimated maximum heart rate.

The body burns a higher percentage of calories from fat in the 'fat burning zone' or at lower intensities. But, at higher intensities, you burn a greater number of overall calories which is what you should be concerned about when trying to lose weight.

Checking Your Heart Rate

To find your heart rate during exercise, slow down enough to take a fifteen second pulse check. You can find your pulse either on the neck or on the inside of your wrist. Then remember to multiply your pulse by 4, because 15 seconds × 4 = 60 sec (bpm).

You can also purchase a heart monitor to measure your heart rate as you exercise.

Many people are warned to stay within their 'fat burning' zone for the best results, but do you really burn more fat if you 0work at lower intensities?

- We burn more calories from fat at lower intensities of cardio, but we actually burn more total calories from fat and more overall calories at higher intensities, done for shorter time intervals.

Will walking help me lose weight?

- Use a pedometer and count your steps. Step counting is a great way to keep active, aiming to increase your steps by 2,000 per day towards a goal of 10,000 steps per day.
- Walking at 2 mph (3.21 kph), a relatively slow pace, burns about 26 calories per 10 minutes. In 30 minutes the average person burns about 79 calories. Picking up the pace and walking about 3 mph (4.82 kph) almost doubles the benefits of a half hour walk. One burns about 125 calories in a thirty-minute period. As one gets more comfortable walking at slower paces, one can begin to burn even more calories by including a few minutes of extra fast walking or jogging to increase heart rate. When one can walk a mile (1.6 km) in 15 minutes, one burns about 370 calories in an hour.

Other Cardiovascular Measurements

- *MET*—1 MET is the amount of oxygen your body takes in when you're not moving.
- MET values tell you how much harder you're working when compared with rest.

So, exercise performed at 3 METs requires three times the oxygen consumed at rest.

- *WATT*—a measure of power; $\dfrac{\text{force} \times \text{distance}}{\text{time}}$

- *Rate of perceived exertion (RPE)*—A person's own perception of the intensity of his or her exercise can be an accurate gauge of exercise intensity. Multiplying the RPE roughly by 10 approximates the heart rate during exercise. Most people should exercise at an RPE between 3 and 6.

BORG RPE Scale[47]

0. No exertion at all
1. Extremely light
2. Very light
3. Moderate
4. _____
5. Strong (heavy)
6. _____
7. Very strong
8. _____
9. _____
10. Extremely strong

You should always be able to catch your breath and speak comfortably while exercising. Feeling effort or slight discomfort is normal during some exercise. However, you should never sense pain.

Physical Activity Calorie Use Chart[48]

The following chart shows the approximate calories spent per hour by a 100-, 150- and 200-pound person doing a particular activity.

Activity	100 lb	150 lb	200 lb
Bicycling, 6 mph	160	240	312
Bicycling, 12 mph	270	410	534
Jogging, 7 mph	610	920	1,230
Jumping rope	500	750	1,000
Running, 5.5 mph	440	660	962
Running, 10 mph	850	1,280	1,664
Swimming, 25 yds/min	185	275	358
Swimming, 50 yds/min	325	500	650
Tennis singles	265	400	535
Walking, 2 mph	160	240	312
Walking, 3 mph	210	320	416
Walking, 4.5 mph	295	440	572

Major Cardiovascular Training Methods

1. Continuous Training Aerobics

Walking, jogging, swimming, aerobics, cycling, intensity 50 to 85 percent.

- *Long, slow distance workouts (LSD)*—increase the number of red blood cells, hemoglobin concentration, muscle capillaries, mitochondrial volume, and aerobic enzymes.
- LSD workouts enhance your muscles' ability to conserve carbohydrates and rely on fat as fuel, so you become a better fat-burning machine.

2. High-Intensity Interval Training (HIIT)

A very high-intensity effort (85 to 100 percent) designed to enhance competitive performance in a specific sport. The best way to lose fat and increase metabolism.

- Involves periods of max or near-max effort followed by short periods of rest. As intensity increases, the contribution from fat is decreased and the contribution from carbohydrate is increased.
- When you exercise at intensity above your lactate threshold, you burn only carbohydrates.
- Short, intense intervals recruit fast-twitch muscle fibers and complement your strength training by adding muscle definition and size.
- Short, intense workouts increase your anaerobic power and capacity by calling on anaerobic metabolic pathways that don't use oxygen.
- Example of short, intense interval-run, cycle, or row at slightly less than all-out pace for 20 seconds to 60 seconds. Takes one to six minutes to recover. Repeat each cycle five to eight times.
- Long aerobic intervals increase the rate at which you consume oxygen by increasing the volume of blood your heart pumps with each beat *(stroke volume)* and the volume of blood your heart pumps each minute *(cardiac output)*.
- Example of long aerobic intervals: run, cycle, or row for two to five minutes at 90 to 95 percent max heart rate, with recovery of two to five minutes. Repeat each cycle three to five times.

3. Circuit Training Methods

Circuit strength training: This workout is a great calorie-burner and perfect for people who want to get more done in a short period of time and burn more fat! Circuit training could be seen as a form of interval training—high-intensity anaerobic bouts of weight training exercises with low-intensity aerobic recovery periods.

The circuit training is comprised of 6 to 10 strength exercises that are completed one exercise after another. Each exercise is performed for a specified number of repetitions or for a set time before moving on to the next exercise. The exercises within each circuit are separated by a short rest period, and each circuit is separated by a longer rest period.

Some sample circuit workouts include:

- Weight circuit—bench press, leg extension, lat pull-down, hamstring curl, bicep curl, squats, tricep extension, and calf raises
- Core circuit—sit-ups, machine crunches, medicine ball, machine back extension, side twists, leg raises, stability ball, flat floor back lifts, and crunches
- Plyometric circuit—jumping jacks, leg kicks, step-ups, jump up into a squat.

4. Circuit Training

Takes the client through aerobic and strength exercises (4–10 stations).

- Each station should be set at 50 to 70 percent of client's functional capacity.

Strength Training Benefits

- Enables muscles to work better
- Capillaries (tiny blood vessels) increase by 50 percent
- Burns fat
- Increases bone density and helps prevent osteoporosis
- Speeds up metabolism and digestion
- Better manage stress and anxiety
- Improves self-esteem
- Improves posture and back pain
- Improves balance

Strength training (and core training): Strength training includes free weights, weight training, plyometrics (jumping jacks, resistance bands), push-ups, sit-ups, and core (torso) exercises. To build muscle, the emphasis should be on higher weight and lower repetitions (6–8) and 3–4 sets. To get cut or look lean, the emphasis should be on lower weight amounts with higher repetitions (8–20), and 2 or 3 sets of several different exercises not lasting more than an hour in total is a general guideline.

In addition, core, or trunk, exercises are some of the most overlooked but most essential supplementary exercises. Core exercises are designed to strengthen your abdomen, your back, and other stabilizer muscles (hip flexors and glutes).

Isometric exercises: Also known as static strength training, this involves muscular actions in which the length of the muscle does not change and there is no visible movement at the joint. Isometric exercises can raise blood pressure significantly for the duration of the exercise. While it will return to a resting level soon after, this can be dangerous for people with hypertension or any form of cardiovascular disease.

Examples of full body isometric exercise:

Plank Bridge

1. Start by lying face down on the ground. Place your elbows and forearms underneath your chest.
2. Prop yourself up to form a bridge using your toes and forearms.
3. Maintain a flat back and do not allow your hips to sag towards the ground.
4. Hold for 10–30 seconds or until you can no longer maintain a flat bridge. Repeat 2–3 times.

Hundred Breaths Exercise

1. Lie face up on a mat with arms by your sides. Bend legs to 90 degrees. Lift your head and shoulders off mat and take 5 short, consecutive inhales, followed by 5 short, consecutive exhales.
2. At the same time, lift arms off mat and pulse them in unison with the breath—palms face up on inhale and down on exhale.
3. Repeat 10 times for a total of 100 breaths.

What Is Your Body Type?

In the 1940s, Dr. William H. Sheldon introduced the theory of Somatypes. His theory described three basic human body types: the endomorph, characterized by a preponderance of bodyfat; the mesomorph, marked by a well-developed musculature; and the ectomorph, distinguished by a lack of either much fat or muscle tissue. He also stated that most people were a mixture of these types.

Ectomorph:

- fragile, thin
- flat chest
- delicate build
- young appearance
- tall
- lightly muscled
- stoop-shouldered
- large brain
- has trouble gaining weight
- muscle growth takes longer

Ectomorphs should concentrate on gaining weight in the form of good lean muscle tissue. Strength training should be fairly heavy and workout pace slower (longer rest periods between sets). Diet should be high in calories (**good quality food, not junk**) and you should eat more frequent meals 5–6 times/day. Aerobic activities should be kept to a minimum, at least until you are happy with your weight gain.

Mesomorph:

- athletic
- hard, muscular body
- overly mature appearance
- rectangular shaped (hourglass shaped for women)
- thick skin
- upright posture
- gains or loses weight easily
- grows muscle quickly

A mesomorph has a naturally fit body, but to maintain it or improve it they should strength-train more often and for longer sessions. You should train with moderate to heavy weights at a moderate pace. If you start getting too bulky, just do lighter weights, more repetitions. A healthy low-fat, higher protein diet will keep you lean and muscular.

Endomorph:

- soft body
- flabby
- underdeveloped muscles
- round shaped
- overdeveloped digestive system
- trouble losing weight
- generally gains muscle easily

An endomorph's biggest concern should be losing the excess body fat. Strength training should be done to get a better muscle-to-fat ratio and to boost metabolism. Endomorphs should eat frequent, small meals—paying attention to the overall calories. Sugars, sweets, and junk food should be eliminated from your diet. Engage daily in some cardio activity.

Working with Weights

Pick calisthenics, free weights, or machine if you intend to work with weights. Just be sure that your strength training includes exercises for every major muscle group, including the muscles of the arms, chest, back, stomach, hips, and legs.

Start with a weight that is comfortable to handle and keep it up for eight repetitions. Gradually add more repetitions until you can complete 12 repetitions. For greater strength conditioning, add more weight and/or more repetitions, in sets of 8 to 12, when the exercise becomes easy.

- *Repetition*—the single performance of an exercise.
- *Set*—a set number of repetitions of the same movement.
- Start with major muscle groups first.
- Maintain proper breathing; exhale on exertion.
- Wait 48 to 96 hours between training the same body part.
- Speed four seconds up, four seconds down.
- To build muscle → decrease reps and increase resistance.
- To tone muscle → increase reps and decrease resistance.
- Change the exercise you perform for each muscle group every four to eight weeks.
- Increase the weight by no more than 10 percent per week.

Why do you need to lift weights in order to lose weight?
- Muscle burns more calories—up to 50 extra calories per pound each day.

Training Frequency[49]
- Beginning: Train entire body two to three days per week.
- Intermediate: Train entire body two to three days per week.
- Split workout: Train each muscle group (upper and lower body) one to two days per week.
- Advanced: Train four to six days per week.
- Elite bodybuilding: Train twice each day for four to five days per week.

Primary Muscle Groups
- Deltoids (shoulders)
- Pectorals (chest)
- Triceps and biceps (back and front of upper arm)
- Quadriceps and hamstrings (front and back of thighs)
- Gluteus maximus (buttocks)
- Trapezius and rhomboids (back)
- Abdomen

Periodization

Instead of doing the same routine month after month, you should change your training program at regular intervals to keep your body working harder while still giving it adequate rest.

For example, you can alter your strength-training program by adjusting the following variables:

- The number of repetitions per set, or number of sets of each exercise
- The amount of resistance used
- The rest period between sets, exercises, or training sessions
- The order of the exercises, or the type of exercises
- The speed at which you complete each exercise

Proper Free Weight-Lifting Techniques

- Warm up before lifting.
- Start slowly and progress gradually.
- Keep weights as close to your body as possible.
- Do most of the lifting with your legs.
- Keep your hips and buttocks tucked in.
- Keep your hands dry or wear gloves.
- Wrap your thumbs around the bar when gripping it.
- When picking up a weight from the ground, keep your back straight and your head level up.
- Use spotters.
- Lower the weights with control.
- Perform all lifts through full range of motion.
- Do not lock the knees or elbows.
- Exhale when exerting the greatest force.
- If you feel pain, stop immediately.
- Stretch and cool down.

Risks of Training

- Overtraining
- Exercise-bulimia
- Injury
- Toxic air
- Congenital defects (hypertrophic cardiomyopathy in athletes)

Signs of Overtraining

- Persistent muscle soreness
- Frequent injuries

76

- Unintended weight loss
- Nervousness
- Inability to relax
- Lower immunity

RICES Concept for Treatment of Injury:
R	Rest
I	Ice application
C	Compression
E	Elevation
S	Support and stabilization

Benefits of Flexibility Training[50]

- Prevention of injuries
- Relief of muscle strain
- Relaxation
- Relief of soreness
- Improved posture
- Better athletic performance
- Improves coordination and balance
- Improves circulation

Factors That Influence Flexibility[51]

- Muscle temperature—Warm muscles stretch more easily than cold muscles.
- Physical activity—Sedentary individuals are less flexible.
- Injury—Injury can limit range of motion; a good rehab program is advised.
- Body composition—Fat can limit movement and flexibility.
- Age—Flexibility declines with advanced age.
- Disease—Arthritis can make stretching painful.

When Performing Any Stretch

- Do a brief warm-up before stretching.
- Start each stretch slowly, exhaling as you gently stretch the muscle.
- Try to hold each stretch for at least 10 to 30 seconds.
- Stretch all the major muscle groups.
- Repeat the stretch four times.
- Stretch *at least* two to three times per week.

Avoid These Stretching Mistakes

- Don't bounce a stretch. Holding a stretch is more effective and there is less risk of injury.
- Don't stretch a muscle that is not warmed up.
- Don't strain or push a muscle too far. If a stretch hurts, ease up.
- Don't hold your breath.
- Do not stretch a swollen joint.

Ways to Improve Posture[52]

- Sit correctly—distribute weight evenly on both hips, do not cross the legs, keep shoulders back and back straight.
- Stand correctly—hold head up, shoulders back, chest forward, stomach tucked in.
- Lift correctly—keep back straight and bend at knees and hips, keep feet wide, lift object using the leg muscles, not the back.
- Lie in bed correctly—lie on your side with your hips and knees slightly bent; put a flat pillow between your knees.

Temperature Extremes

Exercise in Hot, Humid Weather

- Work out in the cooler part of the day.
- Wear light, porous clothing.
- Slow down and shorten your exercise session.
- Drink 12 to 20 ounces of fluid 15 to 30 minutes before exercising and 6 to 8 ounces every 15 minutes during exercise.

Exercise in Cold Weather

- Dress in layers.
- Protect exposed areas.
- Cover your mouth with a mask or scarf on very cold days.
- Wear special cold-weather clothing.
- Drink plenty of fluids.

Safety

- Do not exercise if you are sick.
- Drink plenty of water—remember that thirst is a sign of dehydration.
- Drink 7 to 10 ounces of water for every 10 to 20 minutes of activity.[53]
- Do not exercise if you are sleep deprived.
- Do not exercise if you are fasting.
- Wear the proper clothing and shoes to prevent injuries.

Physical Activity at Home[54]

- Do housework yourself instead of hiring someone else to do it.
- Work in the garden or mow the grass. Using a riding mower doesn't count! Rake leaves, prune, dig, and pick up trash.
- Go out for a short walk before breakfast, after dinner, or both! Start with 5 to 10 minutes and work up to 30 minutes.
- Walk or bike to the corner store instead of driving.
- When walking, pick up the pace from leisurely to brisk. Choose a hilly route. When watching TV, sit up instead of lying on the sofa. Better yet, spend a few minutes pedaling on your stationary bicycle while watching TV. Throw away your video remote control. Instead of asking someone to bring you a drink, get up off the couch and get it yourself.
- Stand up while talking on the telephone.
- Walk the dog.
- Park farther away at the shopping mall and walk the extra distance. Wear your walking shoes and sneak in an extra lap or two around the mall.
- Stretch to reach items in high places and squat or bend to look at items at floor level.
- Keep exercise equipment repaired and in good condition, and use it!

Stay Motivated

- Develop and exercise good habits.
- Reserve a time slot each day for working out.
- Seek support from family and friends.
- Plan ahead and follow your plan.
- Team up with an exercise buddy or consider hiring a personal trainer.
- Set realistic exercise goals.
- Keep an exercise log and make it visible.
- Have fun with your exercise.
- Add variety.
- Affirm your dedication every day.
- Listen to your body.
- Complement exercise with good nutrition.

If You Relapse: How to Get Back on Track

- Look upon every relapse as a learning experience.
- Stop the negative self-talk—*remember that more than half the people who start an exercise program drop out within the first six months.*
- Reevaluate your goals.
- Start performing some kind of exercise *today.*
- Reevaluate your plan.

Thinking of quitting? Make a list of the benefits of sticking to your exercise program and the risks of quitting. Weigh the pros and cons.

_____

_____

_____

_____

_____

_____

_____

_____

When your life gets more hectic, it gets harder to find time to exercise. How can you incorporate exercise into your daily routine so that it's doable? List all the possible exercise "substitutes" you can count on during your busiest times.

_____

_____

_____

_____

_____

_____

_____

_____

_____

_____

Performance-Boosting Drugs

Androstenodione (Andro-DHEA)

- Androstenodione is a testosterone precursor normally produced by the adrenal glands and gonads.

Claims

- Improves testosterone concentration, increases muscular strength and mass, helps reduce body fat, enhances mood, and improves sexual performance

Risks

- Breast enlargement, increased risk of cardiovascular disease and pancreatic cancer in men, acne, male pattern baldness, and a decrease in "good" (HDL) cholesterol
- In women, high testosterone levels can cause increased body hair, deepening of the voice, and other male characteristics

Anabolic Steroids

- An anabolic steroid is a synthetic derivative of the male hormone testosterone that promotes the growth of the skeletal muscle and increases lean body mass.

Claims

- Enhances performance and improves physical appearance
- Reported to increase lean muscle mass, strength, and the ability to train longer and harder

Risks

- Liver tumors, jaundice, fluid retention, high blood pressure, severe acne, aggression, and other psychiatric side effects
- Men: Shrinking testicles, reduced sperm count, infertility, baldness, and development of breasts
- Women: growth of facial hair, changes in or cessation of the menstrual cycle, enlargement of the clitoris, and deepened voice

Creatine

- Creatine is an amino acid made by the body and stored predominantly in skeletal muscle. Creatine serves as a reservoir to replenish adenosine triphosphate (ATP), a substance involved in energy production.

Claims

- Creatine supplements increase muscle stores of the compound, which theoretically allows athletes to work out harder and longer.

Risks

- Water retention, weight gain, muscle cramping, diarrhea, dehydration, electrolyte imbalances, and kidney dysfunction
- No benefit for lower-intensity, longer-duration exercises

Other Drugs

- *Testosterone*—same side effects as steroids.
- *Human growth hormone (HGH)*—used for muscle growth but causes gigantism—abnormal enlargement of joints, jaw, and skull.
- *Amphetamines*—stimulate central nervous system and delay fatigue but can cause chest pains, increases in blood pressure, and addiction.
- *Caffeine*—increases motor activity and delays fatigue but can cause irritability, abnormal heart rhythm, and insomnia.
- *Erythropoetin (EPO)*—increases red blood cells and the ability to transport oxygen to muscles. Side effects include thickened blood, strokes, and heart problems.

Nutrition for an Active Life

Timing of Meals

- You can exercise three to four hours after a large meal.
- You can exercise one to two hours after a small meal.
- Best preexercise foods: high carbs, low fat, low protein.
- Best postexercise foods: high protein, high carbs.

Preworkout

- A few hours before exercise, choose easily digestible low-fat foods with a little protein, which will give you energy to sustain the exercise and keep your blood sugar from dropping.
- Yogurt and fruit; a peanut butter sandwich; cereal and lowfat milk; egg and toast

Postworkout

- About 15–60 minutes after exercise, eat a recovery snack or meal with plenty of fluids and carbohydrates to refuel, and some protein to rebuild muscle.
- Tuna sandwich; grilled chicken and baked potato; whole wheat pasta and turkey meatballs; protein shake or bar

Fluids

- Consume at least 2 cups of fluid 2 hours before exercising and again 15–20 minutes before exercise.
- If the climate is hot and humid, consume 4 to 6 ounces of water or sports drink every 15 minutes.
- After exercise, consume at least 2 cups per pound of body weight lost during the activity.

Sports Drinks[55]

Activities lasting longer than one hour can leave your body wanting more than just water. Sports drinks, which typically contain about 50 to 70 calories per serving, plus vitamins and minerals, are an easy answer to both the fluid and carbohydrate drain that comes from prolonged activity.

You should be able to complete your 30-minute run or 45-minute step class without the aid of additional carbohydrates, especially if your goal is weight loss. How you choose to refuel during a workout depends on your body's reaction to what you put in it. For sessions lasting less than an hour, water is sufficient so long as you consume at least 4 to 10 ounces every 15 minutes.

Energy Gels and Bars

Energy gels are a relatively new alternative to traditional sports drinks or bars. They feel similar in texture to pudding and are easy to eat and easy for your stomach to digest. They typically contain about 70 to 100 calories and may also include caffeine and other ergogenic aids.

Energy bars are eaten more often as a snack than as an energy replacement during exercise. Today, the market is saturated with numerous flavors and types, each with a different ratio of fats, carbohydrates, and protein.

At 110 to 350 (or more) calories each, energy bars also provide extra vitamins, minerals, and fiber, which ups their nutritional value considerably. But eating an energy gel or bar is not enough. You must consume enough fluid to replace what's been lost as well as to help speed digestion.

Personal Fitness Contract

My goals:

_____

_____

_____

_____

My reminder system:

_____

My reward:

_____

My inspiration:

_____

Major milestones:

_____

_____

_____

My weekly workout schedule:

Day	Time	Activity	Place
Sunday			
Monday			
Tuesday			
Wednesday			
Thursday			
Friday			
Saturday			

My signature: date:

Witness: date:

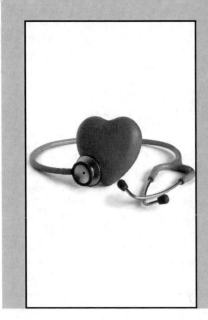

Chapter 5

Chronic Diseases

Chronic Diseases

Heart Disease

Cardiovascular diseases (CVDs) rank as America's number-one killer, claiming the lives of nearly 38 percent of the more than 2.4 million Americans who die each year. Approximately 70.1 million Americans have some type of cardiovascular disease. Cancer follows in severity, killing about 23 percent of those who die each year.[56] Someone dies of heart disease every 35 seconds in the United States.

What Is Coronary Artery Disease?

Coronary artery disease is caused by a narrowing or blocking of the blood vessels that go to your heart. It's the most common form of heart disease. Your blood carries oxygen and other needed materials to your heart. Blood vessels to your heart can become partially or totally blocked by fatty deposits. A heart attack occurs when the blood supply to your heart is reduced or cut off.

Risk Factors for Cardiovascular Disease

Factors You Can Control

Lifestyle factors contribute to the majority of CVD cases in the United States:

- Physical inactivity
- Tobacco use
- Obesity
- Blood fats
- Metabolic syndrome
- Diabetes mellitus

Factors You Can't Control

- Heredity
- Race and ethnicity
- Age
- Gender
- Bacterial infection

Factors

The following nine risk factors account for 90 percent of heart disease diagnosis:[57]

1. *Abdominal obesity* more than doubles heart attack risk in both men and women. Abdominal fat is hormonally active.

2. *Alcohol* acts as a platelet blocker. Modest amounts of alcohol (one or more drinks) reduce a man's heart attack risk by 12 percent and a woman's by 60 percent. Wine has been shown to be highest in protective antioxidants. Too much beer or hard liquor, more than a drink a day, can promote heart disease, cancer, and alcoholism.

3. *Bad cholesterol*—high cholesterol roughly quadruples heart attack risk. It works this way: Bad cholesterol (LDL) carries fats into the artery wall; good cholesterol (HDL) carts it away. A sedentary lifestyle and fatty diet increase LDL and lower HDL. Exercise and a healthy diet switch that ratio and keep arteries clear.

4. *Diabetes* is especially deadly for women, quadrupling their risk of having a heart attack. Men with diabetes double their risk of a heart attack. Like smoking, diabetes causes platelets to stick together, resulting in tiny clots. These clots clog the microscopic blood vessels that feed nerves and arteries, which is a key reason diabetes destroys circulation. Diabetes also raises the level of harmful fats in the blood.

5. *Not eating fruits and vegetables*—eating fruits and vegetables daily cuts heart risk by 30 to 40 percent. Fruits and Vegetables lower bad cholesterol, improve blood sugar, and replace foods that might not be as healthy.

6. *Sedentary lifestyle*—moderate exercise reduces a man's heart risk by 23 percent and a woman's by twice that amount. Exercise improves cholesterol, staves off diabetes by improving blood sugar, and promotes blood vessel growth.

7. *High blood pressure* nearly triples a man's risk of having a heart attack and more than doubles a woman's. Narrowed blood vessels force the heart to work harder, slowly wearing it out. The blood's friction against artery walls also can promote the rupture of plaques, which can lead to heart attacks.

8. *Psychosocial stress*—stressful life events, behavioral disorders, and depression nearly triple heart attack risk. Depressed people with heart disease are four times more likely to have a heart attack or die, and depression is prevalent among 20 percent of people with heart disease in the United States.

9. *Smoking*—smokers are two to three times more likely to have a heart attack than people who don't smoke. Cigarette smoke damages the artery wall, paving the way for inflammation and cholesterol buildup. It narrows arteries. It also activates platelets, sticky cells that cling together and promote clotting. When cholesterol deposits burst inside arteries, clots form.

Facts About Women and Cardiovascular Disease[58]

Misperceptions still exist that CVD is not a real problem for women.

- Cardiovascular disease claims more women's lives than the next six causes of death combined—about 500,000 women's lives a year.

- CVD is a particularly important problem among minority women. The death rate due to CVD is substantially higher in black women than in white women.

- 38 percent of women compared with 25 percent of men will die within one year after a heart attack.

- More women than men die of stroke.
- Low blood levels of good cholesterol (high-density lipoprotein, or HDL) appear to be a stronger predictor of heart disease death in women than in men in the over-65 age group; high blood levels of triglycerides (another type of fat) may be a particularly important risk factor in women and the elderly.
- Diagnosis of heart disease presents a greater challenge in women than in men.
- Women's symptoms are underrecognized, misinterpreted, and sometimes different than men's.
- An apple body shape is more dangerous than a pear shape.
- A sedentary lifestyle contributes to CVD risk.
- Women's heartbeats are faster, thus it takes longer to relax.

How the Heart Works

The normal heart is a strong, hard-working pump made of muscle tissue. It's about the size of a person's fist.

The heart has four chambers. The upper two chambers are the right atrium and left atrium, and the lower two are the right ventricle and left ventricle. Blood is pumped through the chambers, aided by four heart valves. The valves open and close to let the blood flow in only one direction.

The four heart valves are:

1. tricuspid valve, located between the right atrium and the right ventricle.
2. pulmonary (pulmonic) valve, between the right ventricle and the pulmonary artery.
3. mitral valve, between the left atrium and left ventricle.
4. aortic valve, between the left ventricle and the aorta.

Dark bluish blood, low in oxygen, flows back to the heart after circulating through the body. It returns to the heart through veins and enters the right atrium. This chamber empties blood through the tricuspid valve into the right ventricle. The right ventricle pumps the blood under low pressure through the pulmonary valve into the pulmonary artery. From there the blood goes to the lungs, where it gets fresh oxygen. After the blood is refreshed with oxygen, it is bright red. Then it returns by the pulmonary veins to the left atrium. From there it passes through the mitral valve and enters the left ventricle.

The left ventricle pumps the red oxygen-rich blood out through the aortic valve into the aorta. The aorta takes blood to the body's general circulation. The blood pressure in the left ventricle is the same as the pressure measured in the arm.

What Do Your Cholesterol Numbers Mean?

Everyone age 20 and older should have their cholesterol measured at least once every five years. It is best to have a blood test called a *lipoprotein profile* to find out your cholesterol numbers. This blood test should be done after a 9- to 12-hour fast and gives information about your:

- Total cholesterol
- LDL (bad) cholesterol—the main source of cholesterol buildup and blockage in the arteries
- HDL (good) cholesterol—helps keep cholesterol from building up in the arteries
- Triglycerides—free-floating fatty acids in your blood

Total Cholesterol Level	Category
Less than 200 mg/dL	Desirable
200–239 mg/dL	Borderline high
240 mg/dL and above	High

LDL Cholesterol Level	Category
Less than 100 mg/dL	Optimal

HDL Cholesterol Level	Category
Greater than 60 mg/dL	Optimal

Triglyceride Level	Category
Less than 150 mg/dL	Optimal

What Affects Cholesterol Levels?

- *Diet.* Saturated fat and cholesterol in the food you eat make your blood cholesterol level go up. Reducing the amount of saturated fat and cholesterol in your diet helps lower your blood cholesterol level.

  Foods to avoid for high cholesterol/high triglycerides:
  - Full-fat dairy
  - Fatty meats
  - Tropical oils
  - Trans-fats
  - Simple sugars

  Foods to include:
  - High-fiber/whole grains
  - Fruits/vegetables
  - Nuts
  - Legumes

- *Weight.* BMI >25 means you are overweight. Being overweight is a major risk factor for heart disease. It also tends to increase your cholesterol. Losing weight if you are overweight can help lower LDL and is especially important for those with a cluster of risk factors that includes high triglyceride and/or low HDL levels and being overweight with a large waist measurement (more than 40 inches for men and more than 35 inches for women).

- *Physical activity.* Not being physically active is a major risk factor for heart disease. Regular physical activity can help lower LDL (bad) cholesterol and triglycerides, and raise HDL (good) cholesterol levels. It also helps you lose weight. You should try to be physically active for at least 30 minutes on most if not all days.

Things you cannot do anything about also can affect your cholesterol levels. These include:

- *Age and gender.* As women and men get older, their cholesterol levels rise. Before the age of menopause, women have lower total cholesterol levels than men of the same age. After the age of menopause, women's LDL levels tend to rise.

- *Heredity.* Your genes partly determine how much cholesterol your body makes. High blood cholesterol can run in families.

Heart Attack Warning Signs[59]

Some heart attacks are sudden and intense—the "movie heart attack"—where no one doubts what's happening. But most heart attacks start slowly, with mild pain or discomfort. Often people affected aren't sure what's wrong and wait too long before getting help.

- *Chest discomfort.* Most heart attacks involve discomfort in the center of the chest that lasts more than a few minutes, or that goes away and comes back. It can feel like uncomfortable pressure, squeezing, fullness, or pain.
- *Discomfort in other areas of the upper body.* Symptoms can include pain or discomfort in one or both arms, the back, neck, jaw, or stomach.
- *Shortness of breath.* May occur with or without chest discomfort.
- *Other signs.* These may include breaking out in a cold sweat, nausea, or lightheadedness.

> *As with men, women's most common heart attack symptom is chest pain or discomfort. But women are somewhat more likely than men to experience some of the other common symptoms, particularly shortness of breath, nausea/vomiting, and back, abdominal, or jaw pain.*

If you or someone you're with has chest discomfort, especially with one or more of the other signs, don't wait longer than a few minutes (no more than five) before calling for help. **Call 911.** Get to a hospital right away.

Smoking and Heart Disease

- Smoking is the single most significant risk factor for CV disease and peripheral vascular disease.
- Each year smoking causes 250,000+ deaths from cardiovascular disease.
- Active and passive smoking are both detrimental.

How Smoking Damages the Heart

- Nicotine overstimulates the heart.
- Carbon monoxide reduces the oxygen supply to the heart.
- Tars and other smoke residues increase the risk of cholesterol buildup in the arteries.
- Smoking increases blood clotting.
- Smoking causes irreversible damage to the arteries.

What Is a Stroke?

A stroke occurs when the blood supply to a portion of the brain is blocked. Strokes are the third-leading cause of death in the United States.

Risk Factors for Strokes

- Gender
- Race
- Age
- Hypertension
- High red blood cell count
- Heart disease
- Blood fats
- Diabetes mellitus

Warning Signs of Strokes

- Sudden numbness or weakness of the face, arm, or leg—particularly on one side of the body
- Sudden confusion, difficulty in speech or understanding
- Sudden trouble seeing out of one or both eyes
- Sudden trouble walking, dizziness, loss of balance or coordination
- A sudden, severe headache of unknown cause

Diabetes

Diabetes is a serious illness that is increasing rapidly in New York City and around the country. In just the past eight years, the number of New Yorkers with diabetes has doubled. Diabetes is reaching epidemic numbers.[60,61]

- An estimated 800,000 adult New Yorkers—more than one in every eight—now have diabetes.
- Thousands of New Yorkers have dangerous diabetes-related complications.
- New York, perhaps more than any other big city, harbors all the ingredients for a continued epidemic. It has large numbers of poor and obese citizens, who are at higher risk. It has a growing population of Latinos, who get the disease in disproportionate numbers, and of Asians, who can develop it at much lower weights than people of other races.
- One in three children born in the United States in the year 2000 are expected to become diabetic in their lifetimes, according to a projection by the Centers for Disease Control and Prevention. The forecast is even bleaker for Latinos: one in every two.
- Diabetics are two to four times more likely than others to develop heart disease or have a stroke, and three times more likely to die of complications from pneumonia. Most diabetics suffer nervous-system damage and poor circulation, which can lead to amputations of toes, feet, and entire legs; even a tiny cut on the foot can lead to gangrene because it will not be seen or felt.
- Women with diabetes are at higher risk for complications in pregnancy, including miscarriages and birth defects. Men run a higher risk of impotence. Young adults have twice the chance of getting gum disease and losing teeth.

What Is Diabetes?

Diabetes is a disease in which the body does not produce or properly use insulin. Insulin is a hormone that is needed to convert sugar, starches, and other food into energy needed for daily life. The cause of diabetes continues to be a mystery, although both genetics and environmental factors such as obesity and lack of exercise appear to play roles.

Diabetes Causes Serious Health Problems

- Heart disease and atherosclerosis (hardening of the arteries)
- Stroke
- Eye problems and blindness
- Kidney disease
- Poor circulation
- Nerve damage
- Foot and leg problems, which can lead to amputation

- Skin problems (infections, boils, scaly skin, itching)
- Gum disease and other oral health problems
- Erectile dysfunction (impotence) in men
- Depression
- Premature death

Diabetes Often Has No Symptoms

Many people with diabetes have no symptoms, symptoms that develop gradually over months or even years, or symptoms so mild they go unnoticed. Possible symptoms include:

- Frequent urination
- Excessive thirst and hunger
- Weight loss
- Weakness and fatigue
- Nausea and vomiting
- Sudden vision changes
- Tingling or numbness in hands or feet
- Frequent or slow-healing sores or infections
- Recurring vaginal yeast infections in women

Major Types of Diabetes[62]

Type 1 Diabetes

Cause: results from the body's failure to produce insulin, the hormone that unlocks the cells of the body, allowing glucose to enter and fuel them. It is estimated that 5 to 10 percent of Americans who are diagnosed with diabetes have type 1 diabetes. The immune system attacks cells in the pancreas, preventing the production of insulin.

Age of onset: as early as infancy.

Physical condition: normal weight or thin.

Treatment: insulin injections or pump; close monitoring of blood sugar.

Type 2 Diabetes

Cause: results from insulin resistance (a condition in which the body fails to properly use insulin), combined with relative insulin deficiency. Obesity, resulting from an unhealthy diet and lack of exercise, makes cells resistant to insulin. Most Americans who are diagnosed with diabetes have type 2 diabetes. *Overweight and obesity are the biggest risk factors for type 2 diabetes.*

Risk factors for type 2 diabetes include:

- Overweight and obesity
- Lack of physical activity
- Older age
- Family history of diabetes, or prior gestational diabetes

- Low levels of HDL ("good") cholesterol or high levels of triglycerides (fats) in the blood
- Race/ethnicity—African Americans, Latinos, Native Americans, and some Asian Americans and Pacific Islanders are at higher risk

Age of onset: as early as age 6, but typically age 10 and up.

Physical condition: typically overweight or obese.

Treatment: dietary changes; increased exercise; blood-sugar-lowering medication.

Gestational Diabetes (Pregnancy-related)

Gestational diabetes affects about 4 to 7 percent of all pregnant women. About half of these women will develop type 2 diabetes within 10 years. If untreated or poorly controlled, gestational diabetes can harm a developing baby.

Pre-Diabetes

Pre-diabetes is a condition that occurs when a person's blood glucose levels are higher than normal but not high enough for a diagnosis of type 2 diabetes. There are 41 million Americans who have pre-diabetes, in addition to the 20.8 million with diabetes. People with pre-diabetes are 50 percent more likely to have a heart attack or stroke. Unless they take steps to control weight and increase physical activity, most people with pre-diabetes will develop type 2 diabetes.

Prevention of Diabetes (Type 2)

- Maintain a healthy weight. If you are overweight or obese, lose at least 5 to 10 percent of body weight.
- Get at least 30 minutes of moderate physical activity (such as a brisk walk) on all or most days.
- Eat a diet high in fiber, fruits, and vegetables, and low in saturated fats.
- These lifestyle changes can lower the risk of developing type 2 diabetes by up to 60 percent in people at risk.

To Manage Diabetes, Know Your "ABC'S"

People with diabetes can prevent heart and kidney disease, blindness, amputations, and other complications by knowing and controlling their "ABC'S":

- **A**1C (three-month average blood sugar level): *Less than 7 percent.*
- **B**lood pressure: *Less than 130/80.*
- **C**holesterol: *LDL ("bad") cholesterol less than 100.*
- **S**moking: *If you smoke, quit now. (For free help, call the Smokers' Quit Line at 311.)*

Hypertension

Hypertension is known as the silent killer. One in four adult New Yorkers have been told they have high blood pressure. Hundreds of thousands more have it *but don't know it.* It causes the heart to pump harder than normal and wears out the arteries. The pressure of blood against the walls of arteries is recorded as two numbers: the systolic pressure (as the heart beats) over the diastolic pressure (as the heart relaxes between beats). Normal blood pressure is less than 120 milliliters of mercury systolic and less than 80 milliliters mercury diastolic.

Systolic blood pressure (top number): Pressure exerted by blood against the walls of the arteries during forceful *contraction* of the heart

Diastolic blood pressure (bottom number): Pressure exerted by blood against the walls of the arteries during *relaxation* of the heart

Nearly 50 million Americans have high blood pressure. If left untreated, high blood pressure can lead to strokes, heart attacks, and kidney failure. Conversely, controlling elevated blood pressure can cut strokes 35 to 40 percent and heart attacks 20 to 25 percent. Often, dietary and other lifestyle changes are sufficient to keep blood pressure controlled. If not, it may be necessary to add blood pressure medications such as diuretics, ACE inhibitors, beta blockers, or calcium channel blockers.[63] African Americans are more likely than other groups to have high blood pressure.

Why High Blood Pressure Is Dangerous[64]

- High blood pressure means the force of blood is too strong.
- This makes the heart work harder, which causes the muscle to become thick and stiff.
- It also damages blood vessels, which makes it easier for cholesterol and other substances to build up.
- Untreated high blood pressure increases the risk of:
  - Heart disease
  - Stroke
  - Problems with blood vessels and circulation
  - Kidney and eye problems
  - Premature death

What Is a Healthy Blood Pressure?	
115/75 mmHg	Healthy
120–139/80–90	Pre-hypertension
140/90	Hypertension

Preventing High Blood Pressure

- Lifestyle changes
- Losing weight
- Regular exercise
- Dietary approaches to stop hypertension (DASH diet)
- Restriction of daily sodium intake
- Quit smoking—nicotine raises blood pressure and heart rate. If you have high blood pressure and smoke, you more than double your risk of a heart attack.

What Can I Do to Prevent Chronic Diseases?

Making wise food choices, being physically active, and taking medications can help you reach your targets.

Make Wise Food Choices

Many people find that changing what they eat can make a big difference in their blood glucose, blood pressure, and cholesterol levels. Following are several strategies for making wise food choices:

- Eat less fat, especially saturated fat (found in fatty meats, poultry skin, butter, 2% or whole milk, ice cream, cheese, palm oil, coconut oil, trans-fats, hydrogenated oils, lard, and shortening).

- Choose lean meats and meat substitutes.
- Switch to low-fat or fat-free dairy products.
- Eat at least five servings of fruits and vegetables each day.
- Cut back on foods that are high in cholesterol (such as egg yolks, high-fat meat and poultry, and high-fat dairy products).
- Choose healthier fats that can help lower cholesterol, such as olive oil or canola oil. Nuts also have a healthy type of fat.
- Eat fish two or three times a week, choosing kinds that are high in heart-protective fat (such as albacore tuna, herring, mackerel, rainbow trout, sardines, and wild salmon).
- Cook using low-fat methods (such as baking, roasting, or grilling foods or by using nonstick pans and cooking sprays).
- Eat more foods that are high in fiber (such as oatmeal, oat bran, dried beans and peas such as kidney beans, fruits, and vegetables).
- Eat less salt.
- Cut down on calories and fat.
- Be more physically active; strive for up to 30 minutes of aerobics daily.
- Quit smoking.

Cancer

Cancer develops when cells in the body begin to grow out of control. Normal cells grow, divide, and die. Instead of dying, cancer cells continue to grow and form new abnormal cells. Cancer cells often travel to other body parts, where they grow and replace normal tissue. This process, called metastasis, occurs as the cancer cells get into the bloodstream or lymph vessels. Cancer cells develop because of damage to DNA. DNA is in every cell and directs each cell's activities. When DNA becomes damaged the body is able to repair it. In cancer cells, the damage is not repaired. People can inherit damaged DNA, which accounts for inherited cancers. Many times, DNA becomes damaged by exposure to something in the environment, such as tobacco smoke.[65]

Genetics[66]

- All cancers develop because of genetic alterations of one kind or another. An alteration is a change or mutation in the physical structure of a gene that interferes with the gene's normal functions.
- Some alterations that increase the risk of cancer are present at birth in the genes of all cells in the body, including reproductive cells. These alterations, which are called germline alterations, can be passed from parent to child. This type of alteration is known as an inherited susceptibility and is uncommon as a cause of cancer.
- Most cancers are not due to an inherited susceptibility but result from genetic changes that occur during one's lifetime within the cells of a particular organ.

Skin Cancer

Skin cancer is the most rapidly increasing cancer in the United States, with more than 1 million new cases each year. The most likely reason that skin cancer rates are rising is that people are spending more time outdoors. Ozone layer depletion may also contribute. Using SPF lotion consistently and reapplying when necessary prevents damage to the skin.[67]

Warning Signs

- Any change on the skin
  - A new spot
  - A spot changes in size, shape, or color
  - A sore that won't heal
  - A mole or dark-colored growth, especially one that looks crusty, or oozes or bleeds.
- Use the ABCDs:

  A = Asymmetry: Does one half of the mole look different than the other half?

  B = Borders: Are the mole's edges ragged or not clearly defined?

  C = Color: Is the mole more than one color?

  D = Diameter: From edge to edge is the mole larger than 6 millimeters?

Risk Factors

- Personal or family history of skin cancer
- Moles
- Natural blonde or red hair color
- Skin sunburns easily
- History of excessive sun exposure, tanning booths, or sunburns
- Occupational exposure to coal tar, pitch, creosote, arsenic compounds, or radium

Prevention

- Limit or avoid the sun from 10 A.M. to 4 P.M. even on cloudy days.
- When outdoors wear a large hat to shade your face, neck, and ears.
- Wear sunglasses.
- Wear lightweight clothing that covers as much of your body as possible. Don't forget about the tops of your feet!
- Use sunscreen with SPF 15 or higher and reapply sunscreen regularly throughout the day when outdoors. People allergic to PABA should use PABA-free sunscreen.

Breast Cancer

Even though lung cancer and heart disease kill more women each year, surveys show that women view breast cancer as the biggest threat to their health.

Breast cancer occurs when cells in the breast grow out of control. The cells clump together and form a malignant (cancerous) tumor. Most breast tumors are benign, which means they are not cancerous. Benign breast tumors are not life threatening and do not spread outside the breast. Anyone can get breast cancer (including men), but it usually strikes women over age 50. And the risk quickly goes up with age. Women who have a family history of breast cancer have a higher risk.

Symptoms[68]

Breast cancer may have no symptoms in the early stages. But as the cancer grows, the symptoms may include:

- A lump or mass in the breast or the underarm area
- A change in breast size, shape, or color

- A discharge from the nipple
- A change in the feel of the skin covering the breast (the skin could become dimpled, puckered, or scaly)

Some of these symptoms may be caused by other problems. Only a doctor can know for sure. If you have any of these symptoms, talk to a doctor immediately.

How Do You Lower Your Risk of Breast Cancer?
- Cut down on the amount of alcohol you drink.
- Maintain a healthy weight.
- Eat more vegetables.
- Perform monthly breast self-examinations.
- Undergo clinical breast exams (every three years for women in their 20s and 30s, every year for women 40+).
- Get a yearly mammogram (for all women starting at age 40, younger if other factors indicate higher risk).

Testicular Cancer

Testicular cancer is the most common cancer in men 20 to 35 years old.

Risk Factors[69]
- Having had an undescended testicle, a condition in which one or both testicles fail to move from the abdomen, where they develop before birth, into the scrotum
- Having had abnormal development of the testicles
- Having a personal or family history of testicular cancer
- Having Klinefelter's syndrome, a genetic disorder in males caused by having an extra X chromosome
- Being white

Symptoms
- Enlargement of one testicle
- Dull ache in the lower abdomen or groin
- A painless, lump, or swelling in either testicle
- A change in how the testicle feels
- A sudden buildup of fluid in the scrotum
- Pain or discomfort in a testicle or in the scrotum

Prevention
- Monthly testicular self-exams

How Can You Reduce Cancer Risk?
- Stop smoking!
- Stay out of the sun and sun lamps.
- Limit alcohol.
- Exercise.

- Adhere to a healthy diet.
- Watch your weight.
- Be sexually cautious.
- Check your body.
- Avoid environmental carcinogens.
- Know your family history.

What Is Asthma?[70]

Asthma is a chronic disease that affects your airways, which are the tubes that carry air in and out of your lungs. If you have asthma, the inside walls of your airways are inflamed (swollen). The inflammation makes the airways very sensitive, and they tend to react strongly to things to which you are allergic or find irritating. When the airways react, they get narrower and less air flows through to your lung tissues. This causes symptoms like wheezing (a whistling sound when you breathe), coughing, chest tightness, and trouble breathing.

Asthma cannot be cured, but for most patients it can be controlled so that only minimal and infrequent symptoms occur and an active life can be pursued.

Who Gets Asthma?[71]

In the United States, about 15 million people have asthma. Nearly 5 million of them are children. Asthma is closely linked to allergies. Most, but not all, people with asthma have allergies. Children with a family history of allergies and asthma are more likely to have asthma.

Although asthma affects people of all ages, it often starts in childhood and is more common in children than adults. More boys have asthma than girls, but in adulthood, more women have asthma than men.

Although asthma is a problem among all races, blacks have more asthma attacks and are more likely than whites to be hospitalized for asthma attacks and to die from asthma.

What Are the Symptoms of Asthma?

- *Coughing*—Coughing from asthma is often worse at night or early in the morning, making it hard to sleep.
- *Wheezing*—Wheezing is a whistling or squeaky sound when you breathe.
- *Chest tightness*—This can feel like something is squeezing or sitting on your chest.
- *Shortness of breath*—Some people say they can't catch their breath, or they feel breathless or out of breath. You may feel like you can't get enough air in or out of your lungs.
- *Faster breathing or noisy breathing.*

In addition, people with asthma may have:

- Wheezing when they have a cold or other illness
- Frequent coughing, especially at night (sometimes this is the only sign of asthma in a child)
- Asthma symptoms brought on by exercise such as running, biking, or other brisk activity, especially during cold weather
- Coughing or wheezing brought on by prolonged crying or laughing
- Coughing or wheezing when they are near an allergen or irritant

If you have asthma, you need to know what things worsen your asthma symptoms. Then do what you can to avoid or limit contact with these things. For example:

- If animal dander is a problem for you, keep your pet out of the house and/or at least out of your bedroom and wash your pet often, or find it a new home.
- Do not smoke or allow smoking in your home.
- If pollen is a problem for you, stay indoors with the air conditioner on when the pollen count is high.
- To control dust mites, wash your sheets, blankets, pillows, and stuffed toys once a week in hot water. You can get special dust-proof covers for your mattress and pillows.
- To prevent colds and flu, wash your hands often and get a flu shot every year. Children with asthma should get flu shots, too.
- If cold air bothers you, wear a scarf over your mouth and nose in the winter.
- If you get asthma when you exercise or do routine physical activities like climbing stairs, work with your doctor to find ways to be active without having asthma symptoms. Physical activity is important.
- If you are allergic to sulfites, avoid foods (like dried fruit) or beverages (like wine) that contain them.

Scientists do not yet know how to prevent the inflammation of the airways that leads to asthma. Scientists are exploring some theories:

- Babies exposed to tobacco smoke are more likely to get asthma. If a mother smokes during pregnancy, her baby may also be more likely to get asthma. Personal smoking may also cause asthma.
- Obesity may be linked to asthma as well as other health problems.
- Environmental contaminants and pollution may cause asthma.

What Is Thyroid Disease?

Your thyroid is a small bowtie- or butterfly-shaped gland, located in your neck, wrapped around the windpipe, behind and below the Adam's Apple area. The thyroid produces several hormones, but two are key: triiodothyronine (T3) and thyroxine (T4). These hormones help oxygen get into cells, and make your thyroid the master gland of metabolism. The thyroid has the only cells in the body capable of absorbing iodine.

Risk Factors for Thyroid Disease

- Women > risk then men
- Age > 50 years
- A personal or family history of thyroid and/or autoimmune disease increases risk
- Being pregnant or within the first year after childbirth
- Current or former smoker
- Radiation exposure
- Recent exposure to iodine via contrast dye or surgical antiseptic
- Recent neck trauma, biopsy, injection or surgery
- High-stress life events

Hypothyroidism

This condition is when the body does not produce enough thyroid hormones to properly regulate metabolism.

Some causes are:

1. Inflammation of the thyroid glands
2. Surgical removal of the entire or parts of the thyroid glands
3. Iodine deficiency
4. Postpartum
5. Hashimoto's is an autoimmune disease in which the thyroid gland is gradually destroyed by a variety of cell and antibody mediated immune processes.

Symptoms:

- Goiter (abnormally enlarged thyroid gland; can result from underproduction or overproduction of hormone or from a deficiency of iodine in the diet)
- Brittle finger nails
- Thin, brittle hair
- Muscle cramps
- Poor muscle tone
- Joint pain
- Weight gain
- Inability to tolerate cold
- Dry, itchy skin
- Decreased production of sweat
- Constipation
- Depression
- Slow speech
- Developing a hoarse voice
- Decreased libido in men

Treatment options:

- Some affected persons are given desiccated thyroid extract produced from the thyroid of an animal such as a pig.

Hyperthyroidism

This is the condition where there is an overabundance of thyroid hormones in the body.

Some causes are:

1. Graves Disease, which results when the immune system attacks the thyroid gland. When this happens, the gland produces too much thyroid hormone to fight the attack.
2. Thyroiditis, an inflammation of the thyroid.

Symptoms:

- Weight loss
- Hyperactivity
- Hair loss
- Depression
- Excessive sweating
- Shortness of breath
- Chest pains
- Heart palpitations
- Moodiness
- Infertility
- Menstrual problems

Treatment options:

Surgical removal (partial or full) of the thyroid gland, the use of medication, or the use of radioiodine. When radioactive iodine is introduced into the body, it kills or severely damages thyroid cells.

Natural Ways to Treat Thyroid Problems

Diet: Eating foods that are high in iodine such as beetroot, radish, potatoes, bananas, nuts and seafood. Limiting the types of foods that increase thyroid hormones, such as RAW cabbage, broccoli, brussels sprouts, sweet potatoes and lima beans.

Herbs: Some herbs have been found to help control hypothyroidism, such as nettle kelp and bladderwrack, but always consult your doctor before using any herbs.

Exercise: At least 30 minutes of exercise daily is recommended.

Vitamin D: Some amount of vitamin D from the sun is good as it aids in metabolism; or take a supplement.

Date: _____   Name: _____

Create a Family Health Tree

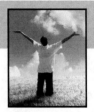

Diseases often run in the family, and knowing your family health history will help keep you healthy.

1. The U.S. Surgeon General operates a free website—go to https://familyhistory.hhs.gov to create a family health history.

   OR

2. Look back into your family's health history. What does it look like? Write down any patterns of diseases or general health problems that run in your family.

_____

_____

_____

_____

_____

_____

_____

_____

_____

_____

_____

_____

_____

_____

_____

_____

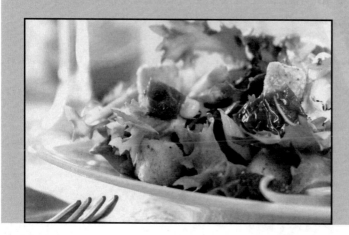

Chapter 6

Nutrition

Nutrition Quiz

Name: _____ Date: _____ Score: _____

In the space provided, mark an F if you think the statement is false and a T if you think it is true.

1. _____ The best diet to lose the holiday weight gain is to eat grapefruits, celery, or cabbage soup.

2. _____ A high-protein/low-carbohydrate diet (Dr. Atkins diet) is a healthy way to lose weight and keep it off.

3. _____ A great breakfast is: 1 glass of orange juice, 1 slice of plain toast, and 1 banana.

4. _____ Starches are fattening and should be limited when trying to lose weight.

5. _____ Bodybuilders, not women maintaining their weight, should eat protein with every meal.

6. _____ Nuts are fattening and you should not eat them if you want to lose weight.

7. _____ Low-fat or nonfat means no calories.

8. _____ Margarine is better than butter.

9. _____ Avoid all candy, including chocolate, to successfully lose weight.

10. _____ Ordering a crispy chicken or cobb McSalad (at McDonald's) is a low-calorie, low-fat alternative.

11. _____ Skipping dinner is a good way to lose weight.

12. _____ Eating after 8 P.M. causes weight gain.

13. _____ "Going vegetarian" means you are sure to lose weight and be healthier.

14. _____ A multivitamin is a great energy booster in the morning.

15. _____ Lifting weights is not a good activity choice if you want to lose weight, because it will make you "bulk up."

> **The only way to keep your health is to eat what you don't want, drink what you don't like and do what you'd rather not.**
>
> —*Mark Twain*

Nutrition

The Six Classes of Nutrients

Macronutrients

- Carbohydrates
- Lipids
- Proteins
- Water

Micronutrients

- Vitamins
- Minerals

■ *Carbohydrates, lipids, and protein contain calories.*

Calorie (kcal) Amount of heat required to raise temp of 1 kg water 1° C. Calories measure the amount of energy that is released when a specific amount of food is burned.

How Many Calories Do I Need?

Multiply your current weight by the following activity conditions:

    14 if you are sedentary

    15 if you exercise 3 times per week; 40 min.

    16 if you exercise 5 to 7 times per week; 40–60 min.

Weight _____ × Activity level _____ = _____ calories/ day

Remember, regardless of whether you consume carbohydrates, protein, or fat, if you take in more calories than your body requires, your body will convert the excess to fat.

Energy Balance

Body fat is a storage tank for energy; to burn body fat you must release energy from storage.

Energy In = Energy Out +/– Fat Storage

1. Energy In > Energy Out = Weight gain
2. Energy In < Energy Out = Weight loss
3. Energy In = Energy Out = Weight maintenance
   - 1 lb. of fat = 3,500 kcals, so if you want to lose 1 lb. of fat per week you need to cut out 500 calories from your daily intake. (500 calories × 7 days = 3,500 calories = 1 lb. fat)

Energy (Calories) Is Needed to Support Three Major Processes

1. Basal (or resting) metabolism
2. Physical activity
3. Growth

Basal metabolism: The sum total of all the chemical activities of the cells necessary to sustain life, exclusive of voluntary activities—that is, the ongoing activities of the cells when the body is at rest.

Basal metabolic rate (BMR):   The rate at which the body spends energy to support its basal metabolism. The BMR accounts for the largest component of a person's daily energy (calorie) needs.

Factors That Affect Metabolism

- Exercise
- Age
- Height
- Yo-yo dieting
- Stimulants
- Frequent meals

How Many Meals Should You Eat Each Day?

Metabolism goes up *only* when you eat consistently all day. You should eat small meals every three hours; divide your total daily calories by 5 to get the number of calories per each meal. For example: 2,000 total daily cal / 5 meals = 400 cal/meal.

Total calories _____ / 5 meals = _____

Goal: Eat five to six small meals per day.

Calorie Values of Common Nutrients

Carbohydrates: 4 calories per gram

Fats (lipids): 9 calories per gram

Proteins: 4 calories per gram

Alcohols: 7 calories per gram

Vitamins, minerals, and water: 0 calories per gram

Acceptable Macronutrient Distribution Ranges (AMDR)[72]

Carbohydrates: 45–65 percent of total daily calories

Fats (lipids): 20–35 percent of total daily calories

Proteins: 10–35 percent of total daily calories

Estimated Calories

Food	Calories	Serving Size
Grains	100	1 slice bread; 1/3 bagel; 1 cup cooked pasta, rice
Dairy	100	1 c. skim, 1% milk; 6 oz. plain yogurt; 1 oz. cheese
Fruit	75	1 piece whole fruit; 1 c. sliced fruit; 6 oz. juice

Food	Calories	Serving Size
Vegetables	25	4 c. salad greens; 1/2 c. carrots, potatoes; 1 c. vegetables
Protein	150	3 oz. fish, poultry, meat; 3/4 c. tofu; 2 eggs; 2/3 c. cooked beans; 1 oz. nuts
Fat	45	1 tsp oil, margarine, butter; 1 Tbsp dressing; 1/7 of avocado
Goodies	100	1/2 c. frozen yogurt; 3 Tbsp ice cream; 4 oz. wine; 2 1/2 oz. mixed drink; 3/4 of a chocolate bar; 2 Tbsp sugar

Some Favorite Meals	Calories
1 c. lasagna; mac & cheese; chili	340
1 c. chicken shrimp w/broccoli	265
1 slice cheese pizza	300
6 pieces sushi roll	225
1 tuna sandwich (homemade)	325
6–8 cheese nachos (no meat)	345
Big Mac & large fries (McDonald's)	1,090
Original Whopper w/cheese, large fries (Burger King)	1,300
KFC 3-piece chicken meal	1,010
Porterhouse steak	1,100
Medium movie popcorn	1,100
Chinese kung pao chicken	1,620

Water

Functions

Water is the most important environmental substance essential to human life. It makes up about 80 percent of the liquid substance of all cells. Approximately 40 to 60 percent of a person's body weight consists of water. Water makes up about 72 percent of the weight of muscle tissue and only 20 to 25 percent of the weight of fat.

- Essential for body temperature regulation
- Transports nutrients and wastes in the body
- Serves as a medium for every enzymatic and chemical reaction
- Maintains blood volume
- Is critical for nerve impulse conduction
- Yields no energy
- Even small amounts of dehydration can impair performance

Goal

64 ounces/day

Proteins

Functions

Proteins are critical for growth, maintenance, and repair of muscles, bones, blood, hair, and fingernails. They are key to synthesis of enzymes, hormones, and antibodies and provide essential amino acids.

Characteristics

- 4 calories per gram
- 22 amino acids total; 9 essential amino acids (must be included through food)
- Complete versus incomplete proteins; may come from animal sources (complete proteins) or plant (incomplete)
- Too much protein = health problems: must be processed (kidneys may be overtaxed)
- In animal form, proteins are associated with saturated fats and cholesterol, heart disease, and osteoporosis.
- You need more protein when you are growing, sick, or injured, have undergone surgery, are pregnant, or are engaging in strenuous exercise.

Dr. Atkins Diet (High-protein, Low-carbohydrate diet)

- Dangerous amount of protein and fat
- Lose water weight, *not* fat
- No energy
- Clogged arteries
- High blood pressure
- Kidney failure
- Ketosis

Smart, Lean Proteins

- Lean chicken—white meat (no skin)
- Fish
- Turkey (white meat)
- Nuts
- Tofu
- Skim milk, low-fat cheese, yogurt
- Egg whites

Goal

0.8–1.0 grams per kilogram

Carbohydrates

Functions

- Provides our brains and body with glucose

Characteristics

4 calories per gram

Simple Carbohydrates (Sugars)

↑blood sugar→↑insulin→fat storage, moodiness, cravings, hunger→quickly absorbs sugar→↓blood sugar.

Simple sugars break down rapidly and the rise in blood sugar provides a quick burst of energy, often followed by a crash.

Monosaccharides (simple sugars) have only single sugar unit in their structure. Monosaccharide units can combine together to form **disaccharides** (containing two sugar units) or **polysaccharides** as starch (containing several sugar units).

- **Glucose**—also known as grape sugar, corn sugar, starch sugar and blood sugar. Found in fruits, vegetables, honey, and starch.
- **Sucrose**—also known as table sugar; is made of glucose and fructose molecules. Found in sugar beets and sugar cane and processed food.
- **Fructose**—also known as fruit sugar. Naturally available in honey; fruits such as apples, pears, grapes, peach, banana, apricot, berries, dried fruits, and melons; and vegetables such as beets, sweet potatoes, sweet corn, carrot, red pepper, onion, yam, and sugar cane.
- **Lactose**—also known as milk sugar. The body breaks lactose down into galactose and glucose.

How to Calculate How Much Sugar Is in a Product

Example: A 20-ounce bottle of Coca-Cola contains about 16.87 teaspoons of sugar. You get this by multiplying 27 (the number of grams of sugar in a serving) by 2.5 (the number of servings in a bottle), which = 67.5 grams of sugar in a bottle. One teaspoon = 4 grams, so divide 67.5 grams by 4 to get the teaspoons of sugar.

What Is Lactose Intolerance?

Lactose intolerance is the inability or insufficient ability to digest lactose. It's caused by a deficiency of the enzyme lactase, which is produced by the cells lining the small intestine. Lactase breaks down lactose, glucose, and galactose, which are then absorbed into the bloodstream. Lactose intolerance is NOT a milk allergy. Milk allergy is a reaction by the body's immune system to one or more milk proteins and can be life-threatening when just a small amount of milk or milk product is consumed.

Symptoms of lactose intolerance:

- abdominal pain
- abdominal bloating
- gas
- diarrhea
- nausea

Two tests are commonly used to measure the digestion of lactose:

- **Hydrogen Breath Test.** The person drinks a lactose-loaded beverage and then the breath is analyzed at regular intervals to measure the amount of hydrogen.
- **Stool Acidity Test.** The stool acidity test is used for infants and young children to measure the amount of acid in the stool.

Treatment

People with lactose intolerance should choose milk products with lower levels of lactose than regular milk, such as yogurt and hard cheese. Lactose-free and lactose-reduced milk and milk products are available at most supermarkets. These products are identical to regular milk except that the lactase enzyme has been added.

Complex Carbohydrates

- Fiber and starch
- Healthier than simple carbohydrates
- Examples: vegetables, grains, cereals, nuts, beans

Goal

- Get at least 130 grams/day to support brain function.
- Limit added sugars to no more than 25 percent of total daily calories.
- Get at least three servings of whole grain per day.

Smart Carbohydrates

- Whole grains
- Oats, wheat, barley, rye, quinoa, couscous
- Brown rice
- Baked potato (with skin)
- Whole-wheat pasta
- Beans
- Whole fruit, *not* juice

Fiber (20–35 g/day)

- Proposed definition (IOM Report, 2001): "consists of non-digestible food plant carbohydrates and lignin"

  Fiber terms:
  - **Soluble:** Makes you feel full; lowers blood cholesterol; beans, oats, carrots, peas, apples, citrus, barley, rice, etc.
  - **Insoluble:** Removes toxins; prevents hemorrhoids, increases elimination; wheat bran

  Both types decrease risk of diabetes, obesity, and certain cancers.

Goal

- *Men:* 38 grams of fiber/day; 50+ years: 30 grams
- *Women:* 25 grams of fiber/day; 50+ years: 21 grams

Fats

Functions

- Carry and help with absorption of the fat-soluble vitamins A, D, E, and K
- Protect organs from injury
- Regulate body temperature
- Play an important role in growth and development

Characteristics
- 9 calories per gram
- Saturated versus unsaturated fats versus trans-fats

Goal
20–35 percent of total daily calories

Saturated Fats
- Increase cholesterol
- Increase LDL
- Increase risk of heart disease
- Increase risk of colon, prostate cancer

  Sources of saturated fat include:
  - Meat, poultry
  - Egg yolks
  - Butter
  - Dairy products
  - Coconut
  - Palm oil

Trans-Fats
- "Partially hydrogenated" or "shortening"
- Produced during hydrogenation of fats in manufacturing
- Increase risk of heart disease
- "Eating plastic"
  - Margarine
  - Baked goods
  - Cookies
  - Crackers
  - Peanut butter
  - Pancake mix

Polyunsaturated Fats
- Lower total cholesterol
- Decrease HDL
  - Omega 3's (fish, walnuts, almonds, flaxseeds)
- Decrease blood clotting and inflammation
- Decrease triglycerides
- Decrease blood pressure
- Decrease risk of heart attacks, strokes, and some cancer

- Slightly increase risk of cancer if Omega 6 consumption is greater than Omega 3 consumption
- Omega 6's (vegetable oils)

Monounsaturated Fats
- Decrease total cholesterol and LDL
- Decrease blood pressure
- Decrease triglycerides
- Decrease risk of heart attacks, strokes, and some cancers
  - Olive oil
  - Peanut oil
  - Avocados
  - Canola

Cholesterol
- Made in the liver
- Only found in animal products
- We need it, but high intake may cause CVD; saturated fats are worse
- Transported in water-soluble vehicles:
  - Very-low-density lipoproteins
  - Low-density lipoproteins
  - High-density lipoproteins

Goal
Less than 200 mg daily

Does Fat Make You Fat?
- The short answer is "yes."
- Carbohydrate stores are limited, but fat is stored in unlimited amounts.
- Excess dietary fat almost always promotes weight gain.
- It is easy to overeat fat—calorically dense, tastes good.
- Dietary fat is easily converted to storage fat.

Smart Fats
- Olive oil, olives
- Canola
- Fish
- Nuts
- Avocado
- Flaxseeds

Nuts

In 2003, the U.S. Food and Drug Administration (FDA) approved this "qualified" health claim on a package label for nuts:

> "Scientific evidence suggests but does not prove that eating 1.5 ounces per day of most nuts, as part of a diet low in saturated fat and cholesterol, may reduce the risk of heart disease."[73]

A "qualified" health claim means the FDA evaluated the data and determined "though there is scientific evidence to support this claim, the evidence is not conclusive." A qualified health claim is issued by the FDA when it is determined that consumers will benefit from more information on a dietary supplement or conventional food label concerning diet and health even though the claim is based on "somewhat settled science rather than just on the standard of significant scientific agreement, as long as the claims do not mislead the consumers." For more information about qualified health claims, go to: www.cfsan.fda.gov/~dms/labqhcqa.html.

According to the FDA, "Types of nuts eligible for this claim are restricted to almonds, hazelnuts, peanuts, pecans, some pine nuts, pistachio nuts and walnuts. Types of nuts on which the health claim may be placed is restricted to those nuts that were specifically included in the health claim petition, but that do not exceed 4 g saturated fat per 50 g of nuts."

Though nuts are a higher-fat food, it is a mostly heart-healthy unsaturated fat and may help lower low-density lipoproteins (LDL or bad cholesterol).

Vegetarian Diets

- *Vegans* exclude all animal products, the most restrictive type of vegetarian diet.
- *Lacto-ovo* vegetarians only exclude meat.
- A modified vegetarian diet promotes health and weight management.
- Legumes and soy have particular health benefits.
- Vitamin deficiencies (protein, vitamin B_{12}, iron, calcium, zinc) can result from a careless vegetarian diet.
- Health benefits of a vegetarian diet include: lower cholesterol, lower body fat, lower blood pressure, and lower risk of some cancers.

Vitamins

Functions

- Help put proteins, fats, and carbohydrates to use
- Essential for regulating growth, maintaining tissue, and releasing energy from food
- Involved in the manufacture of blood cells, hormones, and other compounds

Characteristics

- *Fat-soluble*: vitamins A, D, E, and K; stored in the liver; toxic in high amounts
- *Water-soluble*: B vitamins (eight total) and vitamin C

Antioxidants

- Vitamins C and E and beta-carotene, carotenoids, and flavonoids are antioxidants.
- Antioxidants destroy free radicals in your body.

Free radicals: Result of normal metabolism, pollution, smoking, radiation, and stress

Minerals

Functions

- Help build bones and teeth
- Aid in muscle function
- Help our nervous system transmit messages

Characteristics

- 16 minerals
- *Major:* sodium, potassium, chloride, calcium, phosphorus, magnesium, and sulfur
- *Trace:* iron, zinc, selenium, molybdenum, iodine, copper, manganese, fluoride, and chromium

Goal

- Dietary reference intakes: To find out the dietary reference intake for vitamins and minerals, go to www.iom.edu/.

Phytonutrients

Phytonutrients are substances plants use to defend themselves against disease attacks. These generally colorful compounds, like the lycopene in tomatoes, appear to help humans fend off serious ailments, including cancer and heart disease. They are found naturally in fruits and vegetables.

	Found In	Function	
Vitamin A **Retinol**	liver, fortified milk (Retinol form—see following for carotene sources)	Essential for eyes, skin, and the proper function of the immune system. Helps maintain hair, bones, and teeth.	**Deficiency causes:** night blindness; reduced hair growth in children; loss of appetite; dry, rough skin; lowered resistance to infection; dry eyes **Overdose causes:** headaches; blurred vision; fatigue; diarrhea; irregular periods; joint and bone pain; dry, cracked skin; rashes; loss of hair; vomiting; liver damage
Beta Carotene (pro-vitamin A) (see also vitamin A)	carrots, squash, broccoli, green leafy vegetables	Antioxidant. Converted to vitamin A in the body. (See vitamin A.)	**Claim:** The antioxidant properties of this nutrient may be a factor in reducing the risk of certain forms of cancer.

	Found In	**Function**		
Vitamin D	egg yolk, milk. Exposure to sun enables body to make its own vitamin D.	Helps build and maintain teeth and bones. Enhances calcium absorption.	**Deficiency causes:** rickets in children; bone softening in adults; osteoporosis **Overdose causes:** calcium deposits in organs; fragile bones; renal and cardio-vascular damage	
Vitamin E	corn or cottonseed oil, butter, brown rice, soybean oil, vegetable oils such as corn, cottonseed, or soybean, nuts, wheat germ	Antioxidant. Helps form red blood cells, muscles, and other tissues. Preserves fatty acids.	**Deficiency causes:** rare, seen primarily in premature or low-birth-weight babies or children who do not absorb fat properly; causes nerve abnormalities **Overdose causes:** unknown	**Claim:** The antioxidant properties of this nutrient may be a factor in reducing the risk of certain forms of cancer.
Vitamin K	green vegetables, liver, also made by intestinal bacteria	Needed for normal blood clotting.	**Deficiency causes:** defective blood coagulation **Overdose:** jaundice in infants	

Water-soluble vitamins are not stored in the body and can therefore be consumed daily.

Thiamine Vitamin B$_1$	sunflower seeds, pork, whole and enriched grains, dried beans	Necessary for carbohydrate metabolism and muscle coordination. Promotes proper nerve function.	**Deficiency causes:** anxiety; hysteria; depression; muscle cramps; loss of appetite; in extreme cases beriberi (mostly in alcoholics) **Overdose causes:** unknown, although excess of one B vitamin may cause deficiency of others	
Riboflavin Vitamin B$_2$	liver, milk, spinach, enriched noodles, mushrooms	Needed for metabolism of all foods and the release of energy to cells. Essential to the functioning of vitamin B$_6$ and niacin.	**Deficiency causes:** cracks and sores around the mouth and nose; visual problems **Overdose causes:** see vitamin B$_1$	

	Found In	**Function**	
Niacin **Vitamin B$_3$** Niacin is converted to niacinamide in the body.	mushrooms, bran, tuna, chicken, beef, peanuts, enriched grains	Needed in many enzymes that convert food to energy. Helps maintain a healthy digestive tract and nervous system. In very large doses, lowers cholesterol (large doses should only be taken under the advice of a physician).	**Deficiency causes:** in extreme cases, pellagra, a disease characterized by dermatitis, diarrhea, and mouth sores **Overdose causes:** hot flashes; ulcers; liver disorders; high blood sugar and uric acid; cardiac arrythmias
Pantothenic Acid **Vitamin B$_5$**	abundant in animal tissues, whole-grain cereals, and legumes	Converts food to molecular forms. Needed to manufacture adrenal hormones and chemicals that regulate nerve function.	**Deficiency causes:** unclear in humans **Overdose causes:** see Vitamin B$_1$
Vitamin B$_6$ **Pyridoxine**	animal protein foods, spinach, broccoli, bananas	Needed for protein metabolism and absorption, carbohydrate metabolism. Helps form red blood cells. Promotes nerve and brain function.	**Deficiency causes:** anemia; irritability; patches of itchy, scaling skin; convulsions **Overdose causes:** nerve damage
Vitamin B$_{12}$ **Cyanocobalamin**	found almost exclusively in animal products	Builds genetic material. Helps form red blood cells.	**Deficiency causes:** pernicious anemia; nerve damage. (Note: Deficiency rare except in strict vegetarians, the elderly, or people with malabsorption disorders.) **Overdose causes:** see vitamin B$_1$
Biotin	cheese, egg yolk, cauliflower, peanut butter	Needed for metabolism of glucose and formation of certain fatty acids. Essential for proper body chemistry.	**Deficiency causes:** seborrhic dermatitis in infants; rare in adults, but can be induced by consuming large amounts of egg whites—anorexia, nausea, vomiting, dry scaly skin **Overdose causes:** see vitamin B$_1$

	Found In	Function		
Folic Acid (Folacin)	green leafy vegetables, orange juice, organ meats, sprouts	Essential for the manufacture of genetic material as well as protein metabolism and red blood cell formation.	**Deficiency causes:** impaired cell division; anemia; diarrhea; gastrointestinal upsets; spina bifida **Overdose causes:** convulsions in epileptics; may mask pernicious anemia (see vitamin B_{12} deficiency)	**Claim:** Adequate amounts of this nutrient in the first stage of pregnancy may reduce the risks of neural tube birth defects.
Vitamin C Ascorbic Acid	citrus fruits, strawberries, broccoli, green peppers	Antioxidant. Helps bind cells together and strengthens blood vessel walls. Helps maintain healthy gums. Aids in the absorption of iron.	**Deficiency causes:** muscle weakness; bleeding gums; easy bruising; in extreme cases, scurvy **Overdose causes:** unknown	**Claim:** The anti-oxidant properties of this nutrient may be a factor in reducing the risk of certain forms of cancer. May reduce the effects of the common cold.

Minerals found in organic products are essential for body functions.

	Found In	Function		
Calcium	milk, yogurt, cheese, sardines, broccoli, turnip greens	Helps build strong bones and teeth. Promotes muscle and nerve function. Helps blood to clot. Helps activate enzymes needed to convert food to energy.	**Deficiency causes:** rickets in children; osteomalacia (soft bones) and osteoporosis in adults **Overdose causes:** constipation, kidney stones, calcium deposits in body tissues; hinders absorption of iron and other minerals	
Phosphorus	chicken, breast milk, lentils, egg yolks, nuts, cheese	With calcium builds bones and teeth. Needed for metabolism, body chemistry, nerve and muscle function.	**Deficiency causes:** (rare) weakness; bone pain; anorexia **Overdose causes:** hinders body's absorption of calcium	
Magnesium	spinach, beef greens, broccoli, tofu, popcorn, cashews, wheat bran	Activates enzymes needed to release energy in body. Needed by cells for genetic material and bone growth.	**Deficiency causes:** nausea; irritability; muscle weakness; twitching; cramps; cardiac arrhythmias **Overdose causes:** nausea; vomiting; low blood pressure; nervous system disorders	**Warning:** Overdose can be fatal to people with kidney disease.

	Found In	Function	
Potassium	peanuts, bananas, orange juice, green beans, mushrooms, oranges, broccoli, sunflower seeds	Helps maintain regular fluid balance. Needed for nerve and muscle function.	**Deficiency causes:** nausea; anorexia; muscle weakness; irritability (occurs most often in persons with prolonged diarrhea) **Overdose causes:** rare
Iron (Elemental)	liver, lean meats, kidney beans, enriched bread, raisins. Note: Oxalic acid in spinach hinders iron absorption.	Essential for making hemoglobin, the red substance in blood that carries oxygen to body cells.	**Deficiency causes:** skin pallor; weakness; fatigue; headaches; shortness of breath (all signs of iron-deficiency anemia) **Overdose causes:** toxic buildup in liver and, in rare instances, the heart
Zinc	oysters, shrimp, crab, beef, turkey, whole grains, peanuts, beans	Necessary element in more than 100 enzymes that are essential to digestion and metabolism.	**Deficiency causes:** slow healing of wounds; loss of taste; retarded growth and delayed sexual development in children **Overdose causes:** nausea, vomiting; diarrhea; abdominal pain; gastric bleeding
Selenium	adequate amounts are found in seafood, kidney, liver and other meats. Grains and other seeds contain varying amounts depending on the soil content.	Antioxidant. Interacts with vitamin E to prevent breakdown of fats and body chemicals.	**Deficiency causes:** unknown in humans **Overdose causes:** fingernail changes, hair loss
Copper	liver and other organ meats, seafood, nuts and seeds	Component of several enzymes, including ones needed to make skin, hair, and other pigments. Stimulates iron absorption. Needed to make red blood cells, connective tissue, and nerve fibers.	**Deficiency causes:** rare in adults, infants may develop a type of anemia marked by abnormal development of bones, nerve tissue, and lungs **Overdose causes:** liver disease; vomiting; diarrhea

	Found In	Function	
Manganese	tea, whole grains, and cereal products are the richest dietary sources; adequate amounts are found in fruits and vegetables	Needed for normal tendon and bone structure. Component of some enzymes important in metabolism.	**Deficiency causes:** unknown in humans **Overdose causes:** generally results from inhalation of manganese-containing dust or fumes, not dietary ingestion
Molybdenum	The concentration in food varies depending on the environment in which the food was grown; milk, beans, breads and cereals contribute the highest amounts.	Component of enzymes needed in metabolism. Helps regulate iron storage.	**Deficiency causes:** unknown in humans **Overdose causes:** gout-like joint pain

What Is a Dietary Supplement?[74]

- Any product intended to supplement the diet that contains at least one of these ingredients: *vitamins, minerals, herbs or other botanicals, amino acids, metabolites,* or combinations of these ingredients
- Usually taken in pill, capsule, tablet, or liquid form
- Labeled as "dietary supplement," not for use as the sole item of a meal or diet

Do I Need a Dietary Supplement?

If any of the below apply to you, ask your physician or registered dietitian about taking a supplement:

- Your busy lifestyle keeps you from eating the recommended number of servings from the food guide pyramid
- You are on a very low-calorie weight-loss diet (<1,200 calories daily)
- You are elderly and not eating as much as you should
- You are a strict vegetarian
- You can't drink milk or eat cheese and yogurt
- You are a woman of childbearing age who doesn't eat enough fruits, vegetables, beans, and grains
- You are pregnant or lactating

How Are Dietary Supplements Regulated?

Under the 1994 Dietary Supplement Health and Education Act (DSHEA):

- Marketers are responsible for making sure that their product is safe and that any claims about their products are true.
- All ingredients must be listed on the label.

- Dietary supplements are not regulated for safety or effectiveness before going to market, and do not need FDA approval prior to sale.
- The FDA monitors safety after the product has been marketed; to file a complaint about a dietary supplement, go to: www.cfsan.fda.gov/~dms/hclaims.html.

Bottom Line

- Get nutrients from foods first.
- Foods contain many helpful compounds that are not present in supplements.
- Because dietary supplements are not tested for safety and effectiveness before going to market, some may not contain the ingredients stated on the label.

Dietary Guidelines[75]

Dietary Guidelines for Americans is published jointly every five years by the Department of Health and Human Services (HHS) and the Department of Agriculture (USDA). The *Guidelines* provide authoritative advice for people two years and older about how good dietary habits can promote health and reduce risk for major chronic diseases. The *Dietary Guidelines for Americans 2005* gives science-based advice on food and physical activity choices for health.

What Is a "Healthy Diet"?

The *Dietary Guidelines* describe a healthy diet as one that emphasizes fruits, vegetables, whole grains, and fat-free or low-fat milk and milk products; includes lean meats, poultry, fish, beans, eggs, and nuts; and is low in saturated fats, trans-fats, cholesterol, salt (sodium), and added sugars.

Key Recommendations for the General Population[76]

ADEQUATE NUTRIENTS WITHIN CALORIE NEEDS
- Consume a variety of nutrient-dense foods and beverages within and among the basic food groups while choosing foods that limit the intake of saturated and trans-fats, cholesterol, added sugars, salt, and alcohol.
- Meet recommended intakes within energy needs by adopting a balanced eating pattern, such as the USDA Food Guide or the Dietary Approaches to Stop Hypertension (DASH) eating plan.

WEIGHT MANAGEMENT
- To maintain body weight in a healthy range, balance calories from foods and beverages with calories expended.
- To prevent gradual weight gain over time, make small decreases in food and beverage calories and increase physical activity.

FOOD GROUPS TO ENCOURAGE
- Consume a sufficient amount of fruits and vegetables while staying within energy needs. Two cups of fruit and 2 1/2 cups of vegetables per day are recommended for the referenced 2,000-calorie intake, with higher or lower amounts depending on the calorie level.
- Choose a variety of fruits and vegetables each day. In particular, select from all five vegetable subgroups (dark green, orange, legumes, starchy vegetables, and other vegetables) several times a week.

- Consume three or more ounce-equivalents of whole-grain products per day, with the rest of the recommended grains coming from enriched or whole-grain products. In general, at least half the grains should come from whole grains.
- Consume three cups per day of fat-free or low-fat milk or equivalent milk products.

FATS
- Consume less than 10 percent of calories from saturated fatty acids and less than 300 mg/day of cholesterol, and keep trans-fatty acid consumption as low as possible.
- Keep total fat intake between 20 to 35 percent of calories, with most fats coming from sources of polyunsaturated and monounsaturated fatty acids, such as fish, nuts, and vegetable oils.
- When selecting and preparing meat, poultry, dry beans, and milk or milk products, make choices that are lean, low-fat, or fat-free.
- Limit intake of fats and oils high in saturated and/or trans-fatty acids, and choose products low in such fats and oils.

CARBOHYDRATES
- Choose fiber-rich fruits, vegetables, and whole grains often.
- Choose and prepare foods and beverages with little added sugars or caloric sweeteners, such as amounts suggested by the USDA Food Guide and the DASH eating plan.
- Reduce the incidence of dental caries by practicing good oral hygiene and consuming sugar- and starch-containing foods and beverages less frequently.

SODIUM AND POTASSIUM
- Consume less than 2,300 mg (approximately 1 teaspoon of salt) of sodium per day.
- Choose and prepare foods with little salt. At the same time, consume potassium-rich foods, such as fruits and vegetables.

ALCOHOLIC BEVERAGES
- Those who choose to drink alcoholic beverages should do so sensibly and in moderation—defined as the consumption of up to one drink per day for women and up to two drinks per day for men.
- Alcoholic beverages should not be consumed by some individuals: those who cannot restrict their alcohol intake, women of childbearing age who may become pregnant, pregnant and lactating women, children and adolescents, individuals taking medications that can interact with alcohol, and those with specific medical conditions.
- Alcoholic beverages should be avoided by individuals engaging in activities that require attention, skill, or coordination, such as driving or operating machinery.

Practical Approaches to Healthy Eating

Smart Breakfast Choices
- Oatmeal with walnuts
- Egg-white omelet, one piece toast
- Whole grain cereal, skim milk
- Yogurt with fruit
- Toast with low-fat cheese
- Nutrition bar

- Cottage cheese and fruit
- Other _____

Smart Lunch Choices
- Turkey sandwich, mustard, lettuce, tomato
- Tuna sandwich (low-fat mayo)
- Soup and 1/2 sandwich
- Sushi
- Grilled chicken salad (large)
- Baked potato, salmon
- Other _____

Smart Dinner Choices
- Salad (olive oil, vinegar), meat (3–4 oz.), brown rice (1/2 cup)
- Salad, fish, broccoli, potato
- Salad, chicken/turkey burger or taco
- Salad, chicken/turkey meatballs
- Salad, grilled tuna, mashed cauliflower
- Salad, tofu with vegetables
- Other _____

Smart Snack Choices
- Light yogurt with nuts
- Fruit
- Light cottage cheese
- Peanut butter (1 Tbsp) on apple
- Half sandwich
- Nutrition bar
- One packet oatmeal
- Other _____

Eating for Good Health
- Eat five servings of fruits and vegetables per day.
- Include three servings of whole-grain foods every day.
- Consume a calcium-rich food at each meal.
- Eat less meat.
- Avoid high-fat fast foods.
- Eat small meals.
- Read labels carefully.
- Switch to low-fat and no-fat dairy products.
- When choosing fruits and vegetables, the brighter the better.

- Removing a tablespoon of fat removes about 10 grams of fat and 100 calories—an amount that could represent a 10-pound weight loss in a year.
- The calories in herbs and spices are far less than in breadings, batters, gravies, sauces, and fried foods.

Eating for Increased Energy

- Eat frequently, not in bulk—eating small meals will prevent spikes and dips in your insulin and blood sugar, so you will feel more energy without feeling tired from low blood sugar.
- Control your sugars—eat high-carbohydrate/high-fiber starches, which keep insulin balanced.
- Drink enough water—dehydration will surely make you tired.

Aiming for a Healthy Weight While Dining Out

- Always start with a salad or clear-based soup.
- Resist the pre-meal bread basket or ask to have it removed.
- Share a main dish with a friend.
- Make specific requests: reduced and fat-free dressings; dressing on the side, and so on.
- Request fresh fruit for dessert. Hold the sauce or order red sauces rather than white.
- Inquire about preparation methods. Order steamed, grilled, or broiled dishes instead of those that are fried or sautéed.
- Downsize your order—choose an appetizer or a "small" or "medium" portion.
- Do not eat at an "all-you-can-eat" buffet.
- Take time to enjoy your meal. Chew your food slowly, place the fork on the table in between eating.
- Ask for salad dressing to be served "on the side."
- When your food is delivered, immediately set aside or pack half of it to go.
- Resign from the "clean your plate club"—practice leaving a little something on your plate.

Eating Well on the Run

- Sandwich shop: turkey, fresh sliced veggies in a pita with mustard.
- Rotisserie chicken: chicken breast (remove skin), steamed vegetables.
- Fast food: grilled chicken breast sandwich (no sauce).
- Salad bars: broth-based soups, fresh greens, low-fat dressing.
- Asian take-out: wonton soup, steamed chicken, vegetable mixtures over brown rice.
- Pizza night: choose flavorful, low-fat toppings such as peppers, onions, and broccoli, *not* pepperonis, meatballs, or extra cheese.
- On long commutes or shopping trips, pack some fresh fruit, cut-up vegetables, low-fat string cheese sticks, or a handful of unsalted nuts to help you avoid stopping for sweet or fatty snacks.

Weight-Gain Strategies

- Add extra calories to the milk or juice you drink by tossing in a frozen banana or other fruit and whipping up a smoothie in the blender.
- Try eating more food at each meal. If you normally eat one sandwich for lunch, try eating an extra sandwich.
- Add protein shakes in between meals.

- Lift weights.
- Decrease caffeine and cigarettes.

How to Eat Mindfully

Eating without really even being aware of how much we are eating is called mindless eating. Being mindful is paying attention, on purpose and without judgment, to the internal and external world in the present moment, and so eating with intention and attention. Mindfulness helps you identify the difference between physical hunger and emotional hunger and allows you to self-regulate the quantity of food you eat.

Eating with Intention
Be purposeful when you eat:
- Eat when you are truly hungry.
- Eat to meet your body's needs for fuel and nourishment.
- Eat with the goal of feeling *better* when you finish.

Eat with Attention
Devote your full attention to eating:
- Eliminate or minimize distractions.
- Tune into the ambiance, flavors, smells, temperature and texture of the food.
- Listen to your body's cues of hunger and fullness.

Excerpt from *Eat What You Love, Love What You Eat: How to Break Your Eat-Repent-Repeat Cycle* by Michelle May, MD (Greenleaf Book Group, October, 2009).

Mindful Eating—Eating with Intention and Attention

Exercises for Mindful Eating

1. Turn off the TV, phone, and computer when you are eating.
2. Before you begin eating, look down at your food. Take in what it looks like, how it smells, and think about where it came from.
3. Put a bite in your mouth. Notice how the food feels in your mouth and what it tastes like. Before you swallow, notice the things that happen in your mouth when you put food in. Notice how you salivate, notice the urge to swallow, notice the sensation of chewing.
4. As you swallow your food, notice what that feels like. How does your stomach feel now that it is one bite fuller?

Nutrition-Related Diseases

Osteoporosis

- Osteoporosis is a bone-weakening disease.
- It usually strikes one in four women over age 60, but is diagnosed in young females due to excessive dieting, excessive exercise, amenorrhea, high soda consumption, low body mass index, and cigarette use.

- *Peak bone mass* is achieved at 25–35 years; bone loss begins at age 40.
- *Prevention:* adequate calcium intake and weight-bearing exercise.

Iron-Deficiency Anemia

- "Tired blood"
- Related to too little iron—hemoglobin in the blood
- Usually affects women of childbearing age

Symptoms

- Sensitivity to cold
- Chronic fatigue
- Edginess
- Depression
- Sleeplessness
- Susceptibility to colds and infection

Prevention

- To enhance iron absorption, consume foods high in vitamin C.
- Choose more beans, peas, green leafy vegetables, enriched grain products, egg yolk, fish, and lean meats.
- Don't drink tea with your meals.

Protecting Yourself from Food Poisoning

- Clean food thoroughly.
- Drink only pasteurized milk.
- Don't eat raw eggs (cookie dough).
- Cook chicken and pork thoroughly.
- When shopping, choose meat and poultry last, and don't put them in the trunk. The trunk temperature is too hot and bacteria will grow rapidly.
- Don't let meat sit out for longer than one hour during warm weather. If meat sits out too long, bacteria can produce toxins that can cause illness and stay active even during cooking.
- Refrigerate meat and poultry immediately upon arriving home.
- Purchase ground meat or poultry no more than a day or two before you plan to grill it. Otherwise, freeze them. Grill larger cuts of meat, such as steaks, within four days of purchase or freeze them.
- Completely thaw meat and poultry in the refrigerator or just prior to cooking in a microwave.
- Frozen foods do not grill evenly and may be unsafe. Never defrost on the counter—bacteria will begin to grow. It takes about 24 hours to thaw 5 pounds of meat in the refrigerator.

- Clean up juice spills immediately so a raw product does not get on a cooked product. Juice spills should be cleaned with a paper towel. If using a dishcloth to wipe up raw meat or poultry juices, wash it in hot soapy water before using it again.

- Marinate meat and poultry in the refrigerator. Sauce can be brushed on these foods while cooking, but never use the same sauce after cooking that has touched the raw product.

- Unwashed hands are a prime cause of food-borne illness. Whenever possible, wash your hands with hot, soapy water for 20 seconds before handling food. When eating away from home, pack disposable wipes.

- Cook ground beef patties until brown in the middle and juices are clearish with no pink in them when you cut into the meat (160° F). A hamburger can be brown in the middle and still be undercooked.

- The most accurate way to determine doneness is with an instant-read thermometer.

- Though the USDA recommends ground meats should be heated to 160° F to kill microorganisms, the temperature for a steak can be 145° F for "medium rare." A "medium" steak is cooked to 160° F and a "well done" steak is cooked to 170° F.

- Use a tongs or spatula to turn steaks rather than a fork, which punctures the meat and introduces surface bacteria into the interior of the meat.

- Whole poultry should be cooked to 180° F in the thigh. Breast meat should be cooked to 170° F. When poultry is done cooking, juices will run clear with no pink when you cut into the meat.

- If you're preparing steaks, ground meat, and/or poultry at the same time, use a different knife, utensil, or thermometer to check for doneness. For example, don't use the same thermometer to test steaks as you used for hamburgers. Remember to wash thermometers in hot soapy water and rinse in hot water before and after use.

- Discard any food left out for more than two hours or one hour if the temperature is above 90° F. *When in doubt, throw it out!*

Danger Zone: Between 40° F and 140° F.

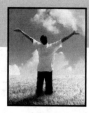

MyPyramid Tracker is an online dietary and physical activity assessment tool that provides information on your diet quality, physical activity status, related nutrition messages, and links to nutrient and physical activity information. The Food Calories/Energy Balance feature automatically calculates your energy balance by subtracting the energy you expend from physical activity from your food calories/energy intake. Use of this tool helps you better understand your energy balance status and enhances the link between good nutrition and regular physical activity. MyPyramid Tracker translates the principles of the 2005 *Dietary Guidelines for Americans* and other nutrition standards developed by the U.S. Departments of Agriculture and Health and Human Services.

One Size Doesn't Fit All

USDA's new MyPyramid symbolizes a personalized approach to healthy eating and physical activity. Want to know the amount of each food group you need daily? Follow the steps below to find out and receive a customized food guide.

1. Go to www.mypyramid.gov.

2. Write a summary of your personalized eating and physical plan.

_____

_____

_____

_____

_____

_____

_____

_____

_____

3. How does your current eating and physical activity compare to the recommendations?

_____

_____

_____

_____

_____

_____

_____

_____

4. Explore your home refrigerator and cabinets. List the foods commonly found in your home. Read and analyze the food labels—look for fat, saturated fat, trans-fat, calories, protein, and sodium content. Analyze at least five different food labels.

_____

_____

_____

_____

_____

_____

_____

_____

_____

_____

_____

_____

_____

_____

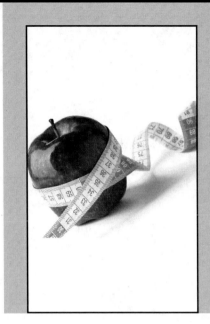

Chapter 7

Obesity and Eating Disorders

What Is Obesity?

Obesity is a disease that affects nearly one-third of the adult American population (approximately 60 million individuals). The number of overweight and obese Americans has continued to increase since 1960, a trend that is not slowing down. Today, 64.5 percent of adult Americans (about 127 million individuals) are categorized as being overweight or obese. Each year, obesity causes at least 300,000 excess deaths in the United States, and health-care costs of American adults with obesity amount to approximately $100 billion.[77,78]

The prevalence of overweight and obesity is increasing worldwide at an alarming rate in both developing and developed countries. Environmental and behavioral changes brought about by economic development, modernization, and urbanization have been linked to the rise in global obesity.

- Obesity is a chronic disease with a strong familial component.
- Obesity increases one's risk of developing conditions such as high blood pressure, diabetes (type 2), heart disease, stroke, gallbladder disease, and cancer of the breast, prostate, and colon.
- Health insurance providers rarely pay for treatment of obesity despite its serious effects on health.
- If maintained, even weight losses as small as 10 percent of body weight can improve one's health.
- The National Institutes of Health annually spends less than 1 percent of its budget on obesity research.
- Persons with obesity are victims of employment and other discrimination, and are penalized for their condition despite the many federal and state laws and policies that ensure equal opportunity.

Leading Sources of Calories in the U.S. Diet

1. Sugared beverages
2. Cake and sweet rolls
3. Hamburgers and cheeseburgers
4. Pizza
5. Potato chips and corn chips

Effects of Modernization

- Rise in car ownership
- Increases in driving shorter distances rather than walking
- Increase in the use of modern appliances (e.g., microwaves, dishwashers, washing machines, vacuum cleaners)
- Increase in ready-made foods and ingredients for cooking
- Increase in television viewing and computer and video game use
- Increase in sedentary occupational lifestyles due to technology and the increase in computerization
- Increase in the use of elevators, escalators, and automatic doors
- Increase in buffet-style restaurants
- Increase in portion sizes
- Higher cost of healthier foods
- More advertisements for unhealthier foods

What Is BMI?

Body mass index (BMI) is a mathematical calculation used to determine whether a patient is overweight.

BMI is calculated by dividing a person's body weight in kilograms by his or her height in meters squared (weight [kg] height [m]^2), or by using the conversion with pounds (lbs) and inches (in) squared as shown below. This number can be misleading, however, for very muscular people, or for pregnant or lactating women.

BMI Table

To use this table, find your weight in pounds across the top row. Follow the column down to meet the box corresponding with your height. The number in this box is your **BMI** (body mass index). Then use your BMI to assess your health risk.

Body Mass Index Table

HEIGHT \ WEIGHT	100	105	110	115	120	125	130	135	140	145	150	155	160	165	170	175	180	185	190	195	200	205	210	215	220	225	230	235	240	245	250
5'0"	20	21	21	22	23	24	25	26	27	28	29	30	31	32	33	34	35	36	37	38	39	40	41	42	43	44	45	46	47	48	49
5'1"	19	20	21	22	23	24	25	26	26	27	28	29	30	31	32	33	34	35	36	37	38	39	40	41	42	43	43	44	45	46	47
5'2"	18	19	20	21	22	23	24	25	26	27	27	28	29	30	31	32	33	34	35	36	37	37	38	39	40	41	42	43	44	45	46
5'3"	18	19	19	20	21	22	23	24	25	26	27	27	28	29	30	31	32	33	34	35	35	36	37	38	39	40	41	42	43	43	44
5'4"	17	18	19	20	21	21	22	23	24	25	26	27	27	28	29	30	31	32	33	33	34	35	36	37	38	39	39	40	41	42	43
5'5"	17	17	18	19	20	21	22	22	23	24	25	26	27	27	28	29	30	31	32	32	33	34	35	36	37	37	38	39	40	41	42
5'6"	16	17	18	19	19	20	21	22	23	23	24	25	26	27	27	28	29	30	31	31	32	33	34	35	36	36	37	38	39	40	40
5'7"	16	16	17	18	19	20	20	21	22	23	23	24	25	26	27	27	28	29	30	31	31	32	33	34	34	35	36	37	38	38	39
5'8"	15	16	17	17	18	19	20	21	21	22	23	24	24	25	26	27	27	28	29	30	30	31	32	33	33	34	35	36	36	37	38
5'9"	15	16	16	17	18	18	19	20	21	21	22	23	24	24	25	26	27	27	28	29	30	30	31	32	32	33	34	35	35	36	37
5'10"	14	15	16	17	17	18	19	19	20	21	22	22	23	24	24	25	26	27	27	28	29	29	30	31	32	32	33	34	34	35	36
5'11"	14	15	15	16	17	17	18	19	20	20	21	22	22	23	24	24	25	26	26	27	28	29	29	30	31	31	32	33	33	34	35
6'0"	14	14	15	16	16	17	18	18	19	20	20	21	22	22	23	24	24	25	26	26	27	28	28	29	30	31	31	32	33	33	34
6'1"	13	14	15	15	16	16	17	18	18	19	20	20	21	22	22	23	24	24	25	26	26	27	28	28	29	30	30	31	32	32	33
6'2"	13	13	14	15	15	16	17	17	18	19	19	20	21	21	22	22	23	24	24	25	26	26	27	28	28	29	30	30	31	31	32
6'3"	12	13	14	14	15	16	16	17	17	18	19	19	20	21	21	22	22	23	24	24	25	26	26	27	27	28	29	29	30	31	31
6'4"	12	13	13	14	15	15	16	16	17	18	18	19	19	20	21	21	22	23	23	24	24	25	26	26	27	28	29	29	30	30

BMI Categories

- Underweight = <18.5
- Normal weight = 18.5–24.9
- Overweight = 25–29.9
- Obesity = BMI of 30 or greater

Childhood Obesity

Prevalence

Obesity in children and adolescents is a serious issue with many health and social consequences that often continue into adulthood. Today's youth are considered the most inactive generation in history, caused in part by reductions in school physical education programs and unavailable or unsafe community recreational facilities.

About 15.5 percent of adolescents (ages 12 to 19) and 15.3 percent of children (ages 6 to 11) are obese. The increase in obesity among American youth over the past two decades is dramatic and due to a variety of causes:

Causes

The causes of obesity are complex and include genetic, biological, behavioral, and cultural factors. Basically, obesity occurs when a person eats more calories than the body burns up. If one parent is obese, there is a 50 percent chance that the children will also be obese. However, when both parents are obese, the children have an 80 percent chance of being obese. Although certain medical disorders can cause obesity, less than 1 percent of all obesity is caused by physical problems. Obesity in childhood and adolescence can be related to:

- Poor eating habits
- Lack of exercise (i.e., "couch potato" kids)
- More TV commercials advertising junk food
- Family history of obesity
- Medical illnesses (endocrine, neurological problems)
- Other

_____

_____

_____

Race

African American, Hispanic American, and Native American children and adolescents have particularly high obesity prevalence.

An American child born in 2000 has a one in three chance of contracting diabetes in his lifetime. An African American has a two in five chance. At current rates, every other Latina born in 2000 will get the disease.

Factors

Modifiable causes of obesity include:

- Physical activity—lack of regular exercise
- Sedentary behavior—high frequency of television viewing, computer usage, and similar behavior that takes up time that can be used for physical activity
- Socioeconomic status—low family incomes and nonworking parents
- Eating habits—overconsumption of high-calorie foods; eating when not hungry, eating while watching TV or doing homework

- Overeating or bingeing
- Medications (steroids, some psychiatric medications)
- Stressful life events or changes (separations, divorce, moves, deaths, abuse)
- Family and peer problems
- Low self-esteem
- Depression or other emotional problems
- Environment—some factors are overexposure to advertising that promotes high-calorie foods and lack of community recreational facilities

In *Food Fight: The Inside Story of the Food Industry, America's Obesity Crisis and What We Can Do About It* (McGraw-Hill, 2003), Brownell cites several factors he thinks give the convenience-food industry an edge in the fight for consumers' taste buds. Unhealthy foods, he argues, are accessible, convenient, engineered with fat and sugar to be tasty, heavily promoted, and cheap. By contrast, healthy foods are less accessible, less convenient, less tasty, not promoted, and more expensive.

Nonmodifiable obesity risk factors include:

- Genetics—Greater risk of obesity has been found in children of obese and overweight parents. If both parents are obese, a child has approximately an 80 percent chance of becoming obese.

Health Risks

- Type 2 diabetes
- Hypertension
- Asthma
- Orthopedic effects
- Psychosocial effects
- Sleep apnea
- Stigma

Prevention

Teaching healthy behaviors at a young age is important since change becomes more difficult with age. Behaviors involving physical activity and nutrition are the cornerstone of preventing obesity in children and adolescents. Families and schools are the two most critical links in providing the foundation for those behaviors.

Prevention Strategies

- Involve the whole family in an exercise program.
- The entire family should eat a healthy diet—together. Eat meals together at the dinner table at regular times.
- Avoid rushing to finish meals.
- Plan special active family-outings such as a hiking or ski trip.
- Assign active chores to every family member.
- Enroll your child in a structured fitness activity.
- Encourage your child in a structured fitness activity.
- Limit the amount of TV watching (<2 hours/day) and move the TV out of the kids' rooms.
- Children should participate in cooking and food shopping.
- Do not watch TV while eating.

- Eat only in the kitchen or dining room—NOT near a TV.
- Avoid foods that are high in calories, fat, or sugar.
- Have snack foods available that are low-calorie and nutritious.
- Watch the portion sizes.
- Avoid using food as a reward or the lack of food as punishment.
- Limit the frequency of fast-food eating to no more than once per week.

Health Effects of Obesity

- Arthritis
- Cancers (breast, esophagus, colorectal, endometrial, renal cell)
- Cardiovascular Disease (CVD)
- Carpal Tunnel Syndrome (CTS)
- Daytime Sleepiness
- Deep Vein Thrombosis (DVT)
- Diabetes (Type 2)
- End Stage Renal Disease (ESRD)
- Gallbladder Disease
- Gout
- Heat Disorders
- Hypertension
- Impaired Immune Response
- Impaired Respiratory Function
- Infections Following Wounds
- Infertility
- Liver Disease
- Low Back Pain
- Obstetric and Gynecologic Complications
- Musculoskeletal or joint-related pain
- Pancreatitis
- Sleep Apnea
- Stroke
- Surgical Complications

Treatment of Obesity

- Dietary therapy
- Behavior modification
- Drug therapy
- Surgery

Dietary Therapy

- Dietary therapy involves instruction on how to adjust a diet to reduce the number of calories eaten.
- Strategies of dietary therapy include teaching about calorie content of different foods, food composition (fats, carbohydrates, and proteins), components of nutrition labels, types of foods to buy, and how to prepare foods.

Physical Activity

- Moderate physical activity, progressing to 30 minutes or more on most or preferably all days of the week, is recommended for weight loss.
- Strategies of physical activity include: the use of aerobic exercise (such as aerobic dancing, brisk walking, jogging, cycling, and swimming), beginning slowly and gradually increasing intensity, and selecting enjoyable activities that can be scheduled into a regular routine.

Behavior Modification

- Behavior therapy involves changing diet and physical activity patterns and habits to new behaviors that promote weight loss.
- Behavioral therapy strategies for weight loss and maintenance include:
  - Recording diet and exercise patterns in a diary
  - Identifying high-risk situations (such as having high-calorie foods in the house) and consciously avoiding them
  - Rewarding specific actions, such as exercising for a longer time or eating less of a certain type of food
  - Changing unrealistic goals and false beliefs about weight loss and body image to realistic and positive ones
  - Developing a social support network (family, friends, or colleagues) or joining a support group that can encourage weight loss in a positive and motivating manner

Drug Therapy[79]

- Drug treatment should be used with appropriate lifestyle modifications.
- Patients should be regularly assessed to determine the effect and continuing safety of a drug.
- Three weight loss drugs approved by the FDA for treating obesity are Orlistat (Xenical), Phentermine, and Sibutramine (Meridia).[80]
  1. Orlistat works by blocking about 30 percent of dietary fat from being absorbed, and is the most recently approved weight loss drug.
  2. Phentermine, an appetite suppressant, has been available for many years. It is half of the "fen-phen" combination that remains available for use. The use of phentermine alone has not been associated with the adverse health effects of the fenfluramine-phentermine combination.
  3. Sibutramine is approved for long-term use, and works to control eating by sending a signal of fullness (satiety) to the brain.

Surgery[81]

- Obesity surgery is recommended as a treatment option for persons with obesity that have: (1) a BMI ≥ 40, or (2) a BMI of 35 to 39.9 with serious medical conditions.
- Obesity surgery is used to modify the stomach and/or intestines to reduce the amount of food that can be eaten.

General Benefits of Obesity Surgery[82,83]

- Weight loss usually occurs soon after obesity surgery and continues for 18 months to two years. Most patients regain some weight after this time, but few regain it all.
- After five years, patients have reported maintaining a weight loss of 60 percent of excess weight.
- Patients will often see improvements in obesity-related medical conditions that they had before surgery, such as diabetes mellitus, glucose intolerance, high cholesterol/triglycerides, hypertension, and sleep apnea.
- Patients have reported an enhanced quality of life, improved mobility and stamina, better mood, enhanced self-esteem and interpersonal effectiveness, and lessened self-consciousness.

General Risks of Obesity Surgery[84,85]

- Some of the complications involve the heart or liver, rupture of blood vessels in the lungs, infection surrounding the diaphragm area, leaking and bleeding of the stomach and intestines, blood clotting of veins, and blockage of the small intestine.
- Other complications include breathing difficulties, wound infections, and injury to the spleen.
- Ten to 20 percent of patients have been reported to need follow-up operations to correct complications such as abdominal hernias.
- Gallstones develop in more than one-third of patients as a result of losing a large amount of weight or from losing weight quickly.
- Anemia, osteoporosis, and other bone disease are nutritional deficiencies that develop after the surgery due to long-term loss of absorptive function.
- Women of childbearing age should be aware that quick weight loss and nutritional deficiencies can harm a developing fetus.
- Pulmonary embolism was the most frequent cause of death in obesity surgery patients.

Types of Obesity Surgery

- *Restrictive surgery*[86,87] uses bands or staples to create food intake restriction. The bands or staples are surgically placed near the top of the stomach to section off a small portion that is often called a *stomach pouch*. A small outlet, about the size of a pencil eraser, is left at the bottom of the stomach pouch. Because the outlet is small, food stays in the pouch longer and you feel full for a longer time.
- *Vertical banded gastroplasty (VBG)* uses bands and staples and is the most frequently performed procedure for obesity surgery.
- *Gastric banding* involves the use of a band to create the stomach pouch.
- *Laparoscopic gastric banding (lap-band)*—approved by the FDA in June 2001, the lap-band is a less invasive procedure in which smaller incisions are made to apply the band. The band is inflatable and can be adjusted over time.
- *Liposuction*—surgically removes fat. This is the most frequent cosmetic operation in the United States.

Eating Disorders

Answer the following questions:

1.	Do you spend time wishing parts of your body looked different?	Yes	No
2.	Are you unhappy with your reflection in the mirror?	Yes	No
3.	Do you skip meals?	Yes	No
4.	Do you count the calories or fat grams in everything you eat?	Yes	No
5.	Do you exercise so much that you are fatigued or have frequent injuries?	Yes	No
6.	Do you avoid eating meals or snacks when you're around other people?	Yes	No
7.	Do you constantly calculate numbers of fat grams and calories?	Yes	No
8.	Do you weigh yourself often and find yourself obsessed with the number on the scale?	Yes	No
9.	Do you exercise because you feel like you have to, not because you want to?	Yes	No
10.	Are you terrified of gaining weight?	Yes	No
11.	Do you ever feel out of control when you are eating?	Yes	No
12.	Do your eating patterns include extreme dieting, preferences for certain foods, withdrawn or ritualized behavior at mealtime, or secretive bingeing?	Yes	No
13.	Do you feel ashamed, disgusted, or guilty after eating?	Yes	No
14.	Do you worry about the weight, shape, or size of your body?	Yes	No
15.	Do you feel like your identity and value is based on how you look or how much you weigh?	Yes	No

What Is Disordered Eating?[88]

Disordered eating is when a person's attitudes about food, weight, and body size lead to very rigid eating and exercise habits that jeopardize one's health, happiness, and safety. Disordered eating may begin as a way to lose a few pounds or get in shape, but these behaviors can quickly get out of control, become obsessions, and may even turn into an eating disorder.

Eating disorders are illnesses with a biological basis modified and influenced by emotional and cultural factors. The stigma associated with eating disorders often leads to individuals suffering in silence.

Anorexia Nervosa[89,90]

Symptoms

- Low body weight (15 percent or more below what is expected for age, height, activity level)
- Resistance to maintaining body weight at or above a minimally normal weight for age and height
- Intense fear of weight gain or being "fat" even though underweight
- Disturbance in the experience of body weight or shape, undue influence of weight or shape on self-evaluation, or denial of the seriousness of low body weight
- Disgust with body size or shape
- Distortion of body size—feels fat even though others tell him he is already very thin

Warning Signs of Anorexia Nervosa

- Dramatic weight loss
- Preoccupation with weight, food, calories, fat grams, and dieting
- Refusal to eat certain foods, progressing to restrictions against whole categories of food (e.g., no carbohydrates, etc.)
- Frequent comments about feeling "fat" or overweight despite weight loss
- Anxiety about gaining weight or being "fat"
- Denial of hunger
- Development of food rituals (e.g., eating foods in certain orders, excessive chewing, rearranging food on a plate)
- Consistent excuses to avoid mealtimes or situations involving food
- Excessive, rigid exercise regimen—despite weather, fatigue, illness, or injury—the need to "burn off" calories taken in
- Withdrawal from usual friends and activities
- In general, behaviors and attitudes indicating that weight loss, dieting, and control of food are becoming primary concerns

Health Consequences of Anorexia Nervosa

- Abnormally slow heart rate and low blood pressure
- The risk for heart failure rises as heart rate and blood pressure levels sink lower and lower
- Reduction of bone density (osteoporosis), which results in dry, brittle bones
- Muscle loss and weakness
- Severe dehydration, which can result in kidney failure
- Fainting, fatigue, and overall weakness
- Dry hair and skin; hair loss is common
- Growth of a downy layer of hair called lanugo all over the body, including the face, in an effort to keep the body warm
- Loss of menstrual periods in postpubertal girls and women

Statistics About Anorexia Nervosa[91,92]

- Approximately 90 to 95 percent of anorexia nervosa sufferers are girls and women.
- Anorexia nervosa is one of the most common psychiatric diagnoses in young women.
- Between 5 and 20 percent of individuals struggling with anorexia nervosa will die. The probability of death increases within that range depending on the length of the condition.
- Anorexia nervosa has one of the highest death rates of any mental health condition.

Emotional and Mental Characteristics

- Intense fear of becoming fat or gaining weight
- Depression
- Social isolation
- Strong need to be in control
- Rigid, inflexible thinking—"all or nothing" attitude
- Decreased interest in sex or fears about sex

- Possible conflict over gender identity or sexual orientation
- Low sense of self-worth—uses weight as a measure of worth
- Difficulty expressing feelings
- Perfectionistic—strives to be the neatest, thinnest, smartest, and so on.
- Difficulty thinking clearly or concentrating
- Irritability, denial—believes others are overreacting to his low weight or caloric restriction
- Insomnia

Bulimia Nervosa[93]

Bulimia nervosa is a serious, potentially life-threatening eating disorder characterized by a cycle of bingeing and purging.

Symptoms[94]

- Regular intake of large amounts of food accompanied by a sense of loss of control over eating behavior.
- Regular use of inappropriate compensatory behaviors such as self-induced vomiting, laxative or diuretic abuse, fasting, and/or obsessive or compulsive exercise.
- Extreme concern with body weight and shape.
- Bulimia nervosa affects 1 to 2 percent of adolescent and young adult women.
- Approximately 80 percent of bulimia nervosa patients are female.
- People struggling with bulimia nervosa will often appear to be of average body weight.
- Many people struggling with bulimia nervosa recognize that their behaviors are unusual and perhaps dangerous to their health.
- Bulimia nervosa is frequently associated with symptoms of depression and changes in social adjustment.

Warning Signs of Bulimia Nervosa[95]

- Evidence of binge-eating, including disappearance of large amounts of food in short periods of time or the existence of wrappers and containers indicating the consumption of large amounts of food
- Evidence of purging behaviors, including frequent trips to the bathroom after meals, signs and/or smells of vomiting, presence of wrappers or packages of laxatives or diuretics
- Recurrent episodes of binge-eating: eating an amount of food that is definitely larger than most people would eat during a similar period of time and under similar circumstances
- A sense of lack of control over eating during binge episodes
- Excessive, rigid exercise regimen—despite weather, fatigue, illness, or injury—the need to "burn off" calories taken in
- Unusual swelling of the cheeks or jaw area.
- Calluses or discoloration on the back of the hands, fingernails, and knuckles from self-induced vomiting
- Discoloration or staining of the teeth
- Creation of complex lifestyle schedules or rituals to make time for binge-and-purge sessions
- Withdrawal from usual friends and activities

Health Consequences of Bulimia Nervosa[96]

- Electrolyte imbalances that can lead to irregular heartbeats and possibly heart failure and death. Electrolyte imbalance is caused by dehydration and loss of potassium and sodium from the body as a result of purging behaviors.
- Inflammation and possible rupture of the esophagus from frequent vomiting
- Tooth decay and staining from stomach acids released during frequent vomiting
- Chronic irregular bowel movements and constipation as a result of laxative abuse
- Gastric rupture
- Weight fluctuations
- Edema (fluid retention or bloating)
- Lack of energy, fatigue

Emotional and Mental Characteristics

- Intense fear of becoming fat or gaining weight
- Performance and appearance oriented
- Works hard to please others
- Depression
- Social isolation
- Possible conflict over gender identity or sexual orientation
- Strong need to be in control
- Difficulty expressing feelings
- Feelings of worthlessness—uses weight, appearance, and achievement as measures of worth

Laxative Abuse

Laxative abuse occurs when a person attempts to get rid of unwanted calories, lose weight, "feel thin," or "feel empty" through the repeated, frequent misuse of laxatives. Often, laxatives are misused following eating binges, when the individual mistakenly believes that the laxatives will work to rush food and calories through the gut and bowels before they can be absorbed. But that doesn't really happen. Unfortunately, laxative abuse is serious and dangerous—often resulting in a variety of health complications and sometimes causing life-threatening risks.

Health Consequences of Laxative Abuse

- *Upset of electrolyte and mineral balances.* Sodium, potassium, magnesium, and phosphorus are electrolytes and minerals that are present in very specific amounts necessary for proper functioning of the nerves and muscles, including those of the colon and heart. Upsetting this delicate balance can cause improper functioning of these vital organs.
- *Severe dehydration* may cause tremors, weakness, blurry vision, fainting, kidney damage, and, in extreme cases, death. Dehydration often requires medical treatment.
- *Laxative dependency* occurs when the colon stops reacting to usual doses of laxatives so that larger and larger amounts of laxatives may be needed to produce bowel movements.
- *Internal organ damage* may result, including stretched or "lazy" colon, colon infection, irritable bowel syndrome (IBS), and liver damage. Chronic laxative abuse may contribute to risk of colon cancer.

Binge-Eating Disorder[97]

Binge-eating disorder (BED) is a type of eating disorder not otherwise specified and is characterized by recurrent binge eating without the regular use of compensatory measures to counter the binge eating.

Symptoms

- Frequent episodes of eating large quantities of food in short periods of time
- Feeling out of control over eating behavior
- Feeling ashamed or disgusted by the behavior
- Eating when not hungry and eating in secret
- The prevalence of BED is estimated to be approximately 1 to 5 percent of the general population.
- Binge-eating disorder affects women slightly more often than men—estimates indicate that about 60 percent of people struggling with binge-eating disorder are female and 40 percent are male.
- People who struggle with binge-eating disorder can be of normal or heavier-than-average weight.
- BED is often associated with symptoms of depression.
- People struggling with BED often express distress, shame, and guilt.

Health Consequences of Binge-Eating Disorder

The health risks of BED are most commonly those associated with clinical obesity. Some of the potential health consequences of binge-eating disorder include:

- High blood pressure
- High cholesterol levels
- Heart disease
- Diabetes mellitus
- Gallbladder disease
- Joint problems
- Abnormal blood-sugar levels
- Difficulty walking or engaging in physical activities
- Fatigue

Emotional and Mental Characteristics[98]

- Recurrent episodes of binge eating
- Eating much more rapidly than normal
- A sense of lack of control over eating during binge episodes
- Eating large amounts of food when not feeling physically hungry
- Hoarding food
- Keeping food and eating in secret—eating alone or in the car, hiding wrappers
- Eating until feeling uncomfortably full
- Eating throughout the day with no planned mealtimes
- Emotional eating—often triggered by uncomfortable feelings such as anger, anxiety, or shame
- Feelings of disgust, guilt, or depression during and after overeating
- Binge-eating used as a means of relieving tension, or to "numb" feelings
- Rigid, inflexible, "all or nothing" thinking

- Strong need to be in control
- Difficulty expressing feelings and needs
- Perfectionist behaviors
- Works hard to please others
- Avoids conflict, tries to "keep the peace"
- Disgust about body size, often teased about their body while growing up
- Feelings of worthlessness
- Social isolation
- Depression
- Moodiness and irritability

Treatment for Eating Disorders[99]

- Psychological counseling must address both the eating disorder symptoms *and* the underlying psychological, interpersonal, and cultural forces that contribute to, or maintain, the eating disorder.
- Typically, care is provided by a licensed health professional, including but not limited to a psychologist, psychiatrist, social worker, nutritionist, and/or primary care physician.
- Nutritional counseling is also necessary and should incorporate education about nutritional needs and planning for and monitoring eating choices of the individual patient.
- Many people with eating disorders respond to outpatient therapy, including individual, group, or family therapy *and* medical management by their primary care provider. Support groups, nutritional counseling, and psychiatric medications under careful medical supervision have also proven helpful for some individuals.
- In-patient care (including in-patient, partial hospitalization, intensive out-patient, and/or residential care in an eating disorder specialty unit or facility) is necessary when an eating disorder has led to physical problems that may be life threatening, or when an eating disorder has reached a level of being a severe psychological or behavioral problem.

Basic Principles for the Prevention of Eating Disorders[100]

1. Effective prevention programs must address:
   - our cultural obsession with slenderness as a physical, psychological, and moral issue.
   - the roles of men and women in our society.
   - the development of people's self-esteem and self-respect in a variety of areas (school, work, community service, hobbies) that transcend physical appearance.
2. Whenever possible, prevention programs for schools, community organizations, and so on, should be coordinated with opportunities for participants to speak confidentially with a trained professional with expertise in the field of eating disorders, and, when appropriate, receive referrals to sources of competent, specialized care.

How to Help a Friend with an Eating Disorder[101]

- *Learn* as much as you can about eating disorders. Read books, articles, and brochures.
- *Be honest.* Talk openly and honestly about your concerns with the person who is struggling with eating or body image problems. Avoiding it or ignoring it won't help!

- *Be caring, but be firm.* Caring about your friend does not mean being manipulated by that friend. Your friend must be responsible for his or her actions and the consequences of those actions. Avoid making rules, promises, or expectations that you cannot or will not uphold. For example, "I promise not to tell anyone." Or, "If you do this one more time I'll never talk to you again."

- *Compliment* your friend's wonderful personality, successes, or accomplishments. Remind your friend that true beauty is not simply skin deep.

- *Be a good role model* in regard to sensible eating, exercise, and self-acceptance.

- *Set a time to talk.* Set aside a time for a private, respectful meeting with your friend to discuss your concerns openly and honestly in a caring, supportive way. Make sure you will be some place away from other distractions.

- *Communicate your concerns.* Share your memories of specific times when you felt concerned about your friend's eating or exercise behaviors. Explain that you think these things may indicate that there could be a problem that needs professional attention.

- *Ask your friend to explore these concerns* with a counselor, doctor, nutritionist, or other health professional who is knowledgeable about eating issues. If you feel comfortable doing so, offer to help your friend make an appointment or accompany your friend on the first visit.

- *Avoid conflicts or a battle of the wills* with your friend. If your friend refuses to acknowledge that there is a problem, or any reason for you to be concerned, restate your feelings and the reasons for them and leave yourself open and available as a supportive listener.

- *Avoid placing shame, blame, or guilt* on your friend regarding his or her actions or attitudes. Do not use accusatory "you" statements such as, "You just need to eat." Or, "You are acting irresponsibly." Instead, use "I" statements. For example: "I'm concerned about you because you refuse to eat breakfast or lunch." Or, "It makes me afraid to hear you vomiting."

- *Avoid giving simple solutions.* For example, "If you'd just stop, then everything would be fine!"

- *Express your continued support.* Remind your friend that you care and want your friend to be healthy and happy.

- *Tell someone.* Addressing body image or eating problems in their beginning stages offers your friend the best chance for working through these issues and becoming healthy again. Don't wait until the situation is so severe that your friend's life is in danger.

Body Dysmorphic Disorder

Body dysmorphic disorder is a type of chronic mental illness in which you can't stop thinking about a flaw with your appearance—a flaw that is either minor or imagined. This disorder has sometimes been called "imagined ugliness."

Treatment can be cognitive behavioral therapy or medication.

Body Image

- People with negative body image have a greater likelihood of developing an eating disorder and are more likely to suffer from feelings of depression, isolation, low self-esteem, and obsessions with weight loss.

Negative body image is:

- A distorted perception of your shape—you perceive parts of your body unlike they really are.
- You are convinced that only other people are attractive and that your body size or shape is a sign of personal failure.

- You feel ashamed, self-conscious, and anxious about your body.
- You feel uncomfortable and awkward in your body.

Positive body image is:

- You feel comfortable and confident in your body.
- You have a clear, true perception of your shape—you see the various parts of your body as they really are.
- You celebrate and appreciate your natural body shape and you understand that a person's physical appearance says very little about their character and value as a person.
- You feel proud and accepting of your unique body and refuse to spend an unreasonable amount of time worrying about food, weight, and calories.

Steps to Increase Positive Body Image

1. Remind yourself that true beauty is not simply skin deep. When you feel good about yourself and who you are, you carry yourself with a sense of confidence, self-acceptance, and openness that makes you beautiful regardless of whether you physically resemble a supermodel. Beauty is a state of mind, not a state of your body.

2. Look at yourself as a whole person. When you see yourself in a mirror or in your mind, choose not to focus on specific body parts.

3. Surround yourself with positive people. It is easier to feel good about yourself and your body when you are around others who are supportive and who recognize the importance of liking yourself just as you naturally are.

4. Shut down those voices in your head that tell you your body is not "right" or that you are a "bad" person. The next time you start to tear yourself down, build yourself back up with a few quick affirmations that work for you.

5. Wear clothes that are comfortable and that make you feel good about your body. Work with your body, not against it.

6. Become a critical viewer of social and media messages. Pay attention to images, slogans, or attitudes that make you feel bad about yourself or your body. Protest these messages: Write a letter to the advertiser or talk back to the image or message.

7. Use the time and energy that you might have spent worrying about food, calories, and your weight to do something to help others. Sometimes reaching out to other people can help you feel better about yourself and can make a positive change in our world.

Resources

- **QCC Counseling Center:** 718-631-6370
- **Live Helpline Hours (PST): 1-800-931-2237** M 11:00 A.M.–3:00 P.M., Tue 8:30 A.M.–5:00 P.M., W 8:30 A.M.–4:30 P.M., Th 8:30 A.M.–5:00 P.M., F 8:30 A.M.–5:00 P.M.
- **North Shore University Group:** 516-663-0333
- **Eating Disorder Group at Holliswood Hospital:** 718-776-8181
- **Eating Disorder Group at Winthrop Hospital:** 516-663-0333

A Declaration of Independence from a Weight-Obsessed World

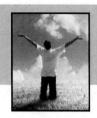

I, the undersigned, do hereby declare that form this day forward I will choose to live my life by the following tenets. In so doing, I declare myself free and independent from the pressures and constraints of a weight-obsessed world.

Initial your name next to each category.

- I will accept my body in its natural shape and size.
- I will celebrate all that my body can do for me each day.
- I will treat my body with respect, giving it enough rest, fueling it with a variety of foods, exercising it moderately, and listening to what it needs.
- I will choose to resist our society's pressures to judge myself and other people on physical characteristics like body weight, shape, or size. I will respect people based on the qualities of their character and the impact of their accomplishments.
- I will refuse to deny my body of valuable nutrients by dieting or using weight loss products.
- I will avoid categorizing foods as either "good" or "bad." I will not associate guilt or shame with eating certain foods. Instead, I will nourish my body with a balance of foods, listening and responding to what it needs.
- I will not use food to mask my emotional needs.
- I will not avoid participating in activities that I enjoy (i.e., swimming, dancing, enjoying a meal) simply because I am self-conscious about the way my body looks. I will recognize that I have the right to enjoy any activities regardless of my body shape or size.
- I will believe that my self-esteem and identity come from within!

_____   _____

Signature   Date

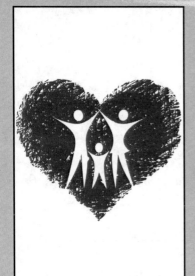

Chapter 8

Relationships and Domestic Violence

Is My Relationship Healthy?

My partner . . .

- Texts me or calls me all the time.
- Get's extremely jealous or possessive.
- Accuses me of flirting or cheating.
- Constantly checks up on me or makes me check in.
- Tries to control what I do and who I see.
- Gets angry and yells at me one minute, and the next minute is sweet and apologetic.
- Makes me feel like I'm "walking on eggshells."
- Puts me down, calls me names or criticizes me.
- Makes me feel like no one else would want me.
- Threatens to hurt me, my friends or family.
- Threatens to destroy my things.
- Grabs, pushes, shoves, chokes, punches, slaps, holds me down, throws things or hurts me in some way.
- Breaks things or throws things to intimidate me.
- Pressures or forces me into having sex or going farther than I want to.

The average age at marriage has risen in most industrial countries. This is due to more women finishing college and entering the workforce. Approximately one-half of the U.S. population is now **unmarried.** People are living together, marrying later in life, or getting divorced.

Define family:

_____

_____

_____

_____

Different Types of Families in the U.S.

The nuclear family was the 1950's scenario of the perfect American household—a heterosexual married couple with two children, a dog, and a white picket fence. After more than fifty years, this perfect family seems to have vanished. Today, families come in all shapes and sizes. Our definition of a family has changed to include different situations like grandparents raising kids, single-parent families, homosexual-parent families, interracial families, adoptive families, and more.

So which is a better environment for bringing up children—a traditional two-parent family or a non-traditional mix we often see today?

_____

_____

_____

_____

Factors Influencing the Change in Family Structure

* More women entering the workforce
* People marrying later on
* Cohabitation
* Easy access to divorce

Divorce

* Approximately half of all marriages end in divorce.
* The younger the couple, the greater the chance of divorce.
* Race and culture affect the rate of divorce.
* The death of a marriage inspires, among other emotions, anger, grief, and fear.

Children and Divorce

Children typically function best when there is routine and stability in their lives. Unfortunately, parental divorce often leads to instability and major change in children's lives. Such changes are associated with a sense of uncertainty and, for some children, uncertainty can lead to feelings of lower self-esteem, poor academic performance, fear, and anxiety and depression.

Studies show that whether or not parents stay married is less important than whether they engage in fighting or conflict—and whether or not they drag the children in. *The critical factor in the ultimate psychological health of a child is the degree of conflict in the environment.*

The decision to divorce is never easy. The painful experience can leave scars on adults as well as children for years. Therefore, before you and your spouse decide to call it quits, consider whether your marriage can be saved.

Issues Couples Cite for Divorce

* Every situation, no matter how seemingly trivial, evolves into a fight.
* You or your partner continually refer to hurtful events in the past.

- All the respect is gone from your relationship.
- Your goals and directions changed while your partner's have stayed the same (or vice versa).
- Your partner is no longer fostering your individual growth.
- You and/or your partner both changed so much that you no longer share moral, ethical, or lifestyle values.
- You and your partner lost the art of compromise. When you disagree you are unable to forge a path together that is acceptable to both.
- You and your partner have a basic sexual incompatibility.
- Other

_____

_____

_____

The Rules of Fair Fighting

"Fair fighting" refers to the technique of "restructuring" couples so that they can fight fairly, learn how to hear the other one through, and do not interrupt, especially to escalate the conflict.

- *Remain calm.* Try not to overreact to difficult situations. Remaining calm will make it more likely that others will consider your viewpoint. Calmly state your feelings about the situation. Talk in a calm, respectful voice. Ranting and raving accomplishes nothing.
- *Don't push one another's buttons.* Don't be sarcastic or attack one another's self-image. Don't interrupt one another.
- *Bar physical and verbal abuse.* Telling someone directly and honestly how you feel can be a very powerful form of communication. If you start to feel so angry or upset that you feel you may lose control, take a "time out"—take a walk, do some deep breathing, exercise, do the dishes.
- *Focus on the present situation.* Past history can raise the emotional barometer; don't bring things up from past fights—focus on the current. Don't stockpile. Storing up lots of grievances and hurt feelings over time is counterproductive. It's almost impossible to deal with numerous old problems for which interpretations may differ. Try to deal with problems as they arise.
- *Be specific about what is bothering you.* Vague complaints are hard to work on. Deal with only one issue at a time. Don't introduce other topics until each is fully discussed. This avoids the "kitchen sink" effect, where people throw in all their complaints while not allowing anything to be resolved.
- *Be flexible and open to other solutions than your own.* Willingness to compromise is important.
- *Avoid clamming up.* When one person becomes silent and stops responding to the other, frustration and anger can result. Positive results can only be attained with two-way communication.

Forming Healthy Relationships

All relationships, whether they are those of parents with their children, spouses with their partners, or workers with their colleagues, rely on an ability to create and maintain social ties.

- Self-esteem
- Friendship
- Trust

- Respect
- Communication
- Compromise
- Support
- Security

Love

Love is defined as an intense feeling of deep fondness or affection for a person or thing.

Three Distinct Stages of Love

1. Lust is driven by the sex hormones testosterone and estrogen.
2. After lust comes attraction. This is the love-struck phase—the time when we lose our appetite, can't sleep, and can't concentrate. When we fall in love, our palms sweat, we stutter and become breathless, we can't think clearly, and it feels like we have butterflies in our stomachs. This is all due to surging brain chemicals called dopamine, norepinephrine, and serotonin. Norepinephrine and serotonin excite us, while dopamine makes us feel happy. These love chemicals are controlled by a substance, which is also found in chocolate and in strawberries, called PEA. Some people become veritable love junkies. They need a constant love high and go through life in a series of short relationships, which end when the initial chemical rush wanes. Love junkies, if they stay married, are likely to seek frequent affairs to fuel their need for the chemical love high.
3. The third stage of love is attachment—staying together. Attachment takes over from the attraction stage and is the bond that keeps couples together. Two different hormones are important during this phase of love: oxytocin and vasopressin. Oxytocin increases the bond between lovers, is one of the chemicals responsible for contractions during childbirth and milk expression when breastfeeding, and is released by both sexes during orgasm. Vasopressin provides a feeling of wanting to be committed to a monogamous relationship.

Toxic Relationships

- Drugs, alcohol
- Violence
- Deception
- Emotional starvation
- Different emotional types
- Unbalanced chores
- Sneaky spending
- Conflicting levels of sexual interest

Codependent Relationships

Codependency occurs when two people form a relationship with each other because neither feels that he or she can stand alone. Codependency is a learned behavior that can be passed down from one generation to another. It is an emotional and behavioral condition that affects an individual's ability to have a healthy, mutually satisfying relationship. Codependents have low self-esteem and look for anything outside of them to make them feel better.

Where does dependency come from? We are born dependent and needy. Becoming independent is the result of a developmental process that involves the support of our parents and other caretakers.

Normal progression begins with *symbiosis*, moves to increasing *competence*, then to *independence*, and, finally to *interdependence*. In codependent relationships, this sequence gets broken, leading to an incomplete sense of self and an inability to become independent.

Symbiosis. In this stage, an infant bonds with its mother and other caretakers.

Competence. The individual develops some ability to be a separate person and to care for him- or herself. As infants become toddlers, they can stand on their own two feet, walk, talk, assert themselves, and grab food from the cabinet.

Independence. Toddlers become children who can make some decisions about what they want. They can dress themselves or are encouraged to make other decisions. Children who are encouraged to make independent decisions and to deal with the consequences of their decisions can begin to feel in control of their lives.

Interdependence. In this stage, children can move comfortably between being both independent and dependent, competent and needy depending on the situation and their own level of growth. It is important for children to know that they can ask for help and support when it is needed without being shamed.

Codependency could result from any of these stages being interrupted, the death of a parent, the breakup of the family, illness, a move, or a traumatic event—all of which intrude on the normal developmental process. Codependency can also result from any of these stages not being supported by parents, other caregivers, and partners who struggle with their own codependency issues.

Dysfunctional Families and Codependency

A dysfunctional family is one in which members suffer from fear, anger, pain, or shame that is ignored or denied. Underlying problems may include any of the following:

- An addiction by a family member to drugs, alcohol, relationships, work, food, sex, or gambling
- The existence of physical, emotional, or sexual abuse
- The presence of a family member suffering from a chronic mental or physical illness

Dysfunctional families do not acknowledge that problems exist. They don't talk about them or confront them. As a result, family members learn to repress emotions and disregard their own needs.

How Is Codependency Treated?

Because codependency is usually rooted in a person's childhood, treatment often involves exploration into early childhood issues and their relationship to current destructive behavior patterns. Treatment includes education, experiential groups, and individual and group therapy. Treatment also focuses on helping patients get in touch with feelings that have been buried during childhood as well as reconstructing family dynamics.

Domestic Violence

Domestic violence can happen to individuals of any race, age, sexual orientation, religion, or gender. It can happen to couples who are married, living together, or dating. Domestic violence affects people of all socioeconomic backgrounds and education levels.

Power and Control

Domestic violence is a pattern of behavior used by an individual to establish and maintain coercive control over his intimate partner.

Statistics

- Approximately 4 million American women experience a serious assault by a partner during an average 12 month period.[102]
- One in four women will experience domestic violence during her lifetime.[103]
- Young women between the ages of 16 and 24 experience the highest rate of domestic violence.
- On the average, more than three women are murdered by their husbands or boyfriends every day.[104]
- One out of three women worldwide has been beaten, coerced into sex, or otherwise abused during her lifetime.[105]
- One in five female high school students report being physically and/or sexually abused by a dating partner. Abused girls are significantly more likely to get involved in other risky behaviors. They are four to six times more likely to get pregnant and eight to nine times more likely to have tried to commit suicide.[106]
- One in three teens reports knowing a friend or peer who has been hit, punched, slapped, choked, or physically hurt by his or her partner.[107]
- For 30 percent of women who experience abuse, the first incident occurs during pregnancy.[108]

Dating Violence and Abuse

Ten Warning Signs of Violence or Abuse

These are ten of the most common, although there are many more signs:

1. Checking your cell phone or email without permission
2. Constant put-downs
3. Extreme jealousy or insecurity
4. Explosive temper
5. Financial control
6. Isolating you from family or friends
7. Mood swings
8. Physically hurting you in any way
9. Possessiveness
10. Telling you what to do

Abuse is a pattern of coercive control that one person exercises over another. *Battering* is a behavior that physically harms, arouses fear, prevents a partner from doing what they wish, or forces them to behave in ways they do not want. Battering includes the use of physical and sexual violence, threats and intimidation, emotional abuse, and economic deprivation.

- Calling bad names or putting someone down
- Shouting and cursing
- Hitting, slapping and/or pushing
- Making threats of any kind
- Jealously and suspicion
- Keeping someone away from family and friends
- Throwing things around the house

Teens who abuse their girlfriends or boyfriends behave similarly to adults who abuse their partners. Teen dating violence is just as serious as adult domestic violence. Teens are seriously at risk for dating violence. Research shows that physical or sexual abuse is a part of one in three high school relationships.

In 95 percent of abusive relationships, men abuse women. However, young women can be violent, and young men can also be victims.

You may be in an emotionally abusive relationship if your partner:[109,110]

- calls you names, insults you, or continually criticizes you.
- does not trust you and acts jealous or possessive.
- tries to isolate you from family or friends.
- monitors where you go, who you call, and who you spend time with.
- does not want you to work.
- controls finances or refuses to share money.
- punishes you by withholding affection.
- expects you to ask permission.
- threatens to hurt you, the children, your family, or your pets.
- humiliates you in any way.
- damages property when angry (throws objects, punches walls, kicked doors, etc.).
- has pushed, slapped, bitten, kicked, or choked you.
- has abandoned you in a dangerous or unfamiliar place.
- has scared you by driving recklessly.
- has used a weapon to threaten or hurt you.
- has forced you to leave your home.
- has trapped you in your home or kept you from leaving.
- has prevented you from calling police or seeking medical attention.
- has hurt your children.
- has used physical force in sexual situations.

You may be in a sexually abusive relationship if your partner:[111]

- views women as objects and believes in rigid gender roles.
- accuses you of cheating or is often jealous of your outside relationships.
- wants you to dress in a sexual way.
- insults you in sexual ways or calls you sexual names.
- has ever forced or manipulated you into to having sex or performing sexual acts.
- has held you down during sex.
- has demanded sex when you were sick, tired, or after beating you.
- has hurt you with weapons or objects during sex.
- has involved other people in sexual activities with you.
- ignores your feelings regarding sex.

Cycle of Violence[112]

Phase I: Tension Building

- Abuser starts to get angry.
- Abuse may begin.

- A breakdown of communication occurs.
- Victim feels the need to keep the abuser calm.
- Tension becomes too much.
- Victim feels like he or she is "walking on egg shells."

The victim may:

- feel like she or he is walking on eggshells.
- try to reason with the batterer.
- try to calm the batterer.
- try to appease the batterer.
- keep silent, try to keep children quiet.
- feel afraid or anxious.

Phase II: Explosion

- Verbal abuse
- Emotional assault
- Sexual assault
- Physical abuse
- Increase control over money
- Destroy property, phone

The victim may:

- experience fear, shock.
- use self-defense.
- call for help.
- try to flee, leave.
- pray for it to stop.
- do what is necessary to survive.

Phase III: Honeymoon

- Abuser may apologize for abuse.
- Abuser may promise it will never happen again.
- Abuser may blame the victim for causing the abuse.
- Abuser may deny abuse took place or say it was not as bad as the victim claims.

The victim may:

- feel forgiveness.
- return home.
- feel hopeful.
- blame self.
- minimize or deny abuse.

The cycle can happen hundreds of times in an abusive relationship. Each stage lasts a different amount of time in individuals relationships. The total cycle can take anywhere from a few hours to a year or more to complete.

The cycle always repeats itself—unless there is an intervention.

Why Does the Victim Stay?

Fear: The number one reason for not leaving is fear.

Lack of resources: Because one of the major components of abuse is isolation, the battered partner most often lacks a support system. Her family ties and friendships have been destroyed, leaving her psychologically and financially dependent on the abusive partner. Economic dependence on the abuser is a very real reason for remaining in the relationship. Public assistance programs have been drastically reduced and those that remain provide inadequate benefits.

Children: Being a single parent is a strenuous experience under the best of circumstances, and for most battered women, conditions are far from the best. Often, the abuser may threaten to take the children away from her if she even attempts to leave.

Feelings of guilt: The woman may believe that her husband is "sick" and/or needs her help; the idea of leaving can thus produce feelings of guilt.

Promises of reform: As is consistent with the cycle of violence the abuser promises it will never happen again; the victim wants to believe this is true.

Religious/cultural beliefs and values: Religious beliefs reinforce the commitment to marriage. Many faiths hold that the husband is head of the family and it is a wife's duty to be submissive to him. This may be a powerful reason for staying in a destructive relationship.

Love for spouse: Most people enter a relationship for love, and that emotion does not simply disappear easily or in the face of difficulty. After a battering, the abuser often is extremely vulnerable. Because her self-esteem is so low following the incident, the apologies and promises of reform are often perceived as the end of the abuse.

National Domestic Violence Hotline: 1-800-799-SAFE (7233)

If you are the victim of domestic violence, the police and courts can help.

The police and the courts can help you get to a safe place away from the violence and help you get an Order of Protection.

An "Order of Protection," sometimes called a "Restraining Order," is an order from either the Family, Criminal, or Supreme Court that orders an abuser to stop committing offenses against you.

Get help now—Get safe—Call:

- **1-800-942-6906 (English) (24 hrs.) or 1-800-942-6908 (Spanish) (24 hrs.)**
- **In New York City, call the all-language 24-hour Domestic Violence Hotline 1-800-621-4673 (TTY 1-800-810-7444) or 311**
- **Victim Information and Notification Everyday (VINE). Victims may receive information relating to the status and release dates of persons incarcerated in state prison or local jails in New York State. For more information on this program and how you can register, call 1-888-VINE-4NY (1-888-846-3469).**

To contact Break the Cycle, call (888) 988-TEEN or www.thesafespace.org

How to Help a Friend in an Abusive Relationship

- Support. Don't judge. Listen.
- If you notice signs of abuse, don't ignore it.
- Talk to your friend about it in private. Don't confront him or her in a public place. Let him or her know you are there for support.

- Express your concerns. Cite specific examples of when you witnessed abuse.
- Tell your friend that he or she deserves better and that the abuse is not his or her fault.
- Don't spread gossip. Honor and protect confidences.
- Don't try to force your friend to do anything he or she does not want to do. Let friends make their own decisions.
- Help your friend take action. Offer to get information for your friend, assist your friend in developing a plan, help your friend find and talk to a supportive adult, find the number for a crisis hotline, and so on.
- Don't carry the burden alone. Encourage your friend to confide in a trusted adult.
- Call the police if you witness an assault.

To help stop domestic violence in your community, call 1-800-END-ABUSE.

Sexual assault and abuse is any type of sexual activity that you do not agree to, including:
- Inappropriate touching
- Vaginal, anal, or oral penetration
- Sexual intercourse that you say no to
- Rape
- Attempted rape
- Child molestation

Rape is a common form of sexual assault. It is committed in many situations—on a date, by a friend or an acquaintance, or when you think you are alone.

Statistics
- Approximately 1 in 5 women and 1 in 33 men have experienced an attempted or completed rape.[113]
- Marital rape accounts for 25 percent of all rapes, affecting over 75,000 women each year.[114]
- Three in four women over age 18 who reported being raped were physically assaulted by a current or former husband, boyfriend, or date.[115]

If You've Been Sexually Assaulted[116]
- Get away from the attacker to a safe place as fast as you can. Then call 9-1-1 or the police.
- Call a friend or family member you trust. You also can call a crisis center or a hotline to talk with a counselor. One hotline is the **National Sexual Assault Hotline at 800-656-HOPE (4673).** Feelings of shame, guilt, fear, and shock are normal. It is important to get counseling from a trusted professional.
- Do not wash, comb, or clean any part of your body. Do not change clothes if possible, so the hospital staff can collect evidence. Do not touch or change anything at the scene of the assault.
- Go to your nearest hospital emergency room as soon as possible. You need to be examined, treated for any injuries, and screened for possible sexually transmitted diseases (STDs) or pregnancy. The doctor will collect evidence using a rape kit for fibers, hairs, saliva, semen, or clothing that the attacker may have left behind.
- You or the hospital staff can call the police from the emergency room to file a report.
- Ask the hospital staff about possible support groups you can attend right away.

Safety During a Violent Incident

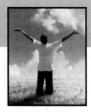

Victims cannot always avoid violent incidents. In order to increase safety, victims may use a variety of strategies.

If violence reoccurs or if you are afraid that the violence will reoccur, you can enhance your safety by creating an action plan such as the following:

When I have to communicate with my partner/abuser in person or by telephone and he or she becomes abusive, I can

_____

_____

_____

When I have contact with my abuser at my home and I expect we are going to have an argument, I will try to move to a space that is lowest risk, such as _____. (Try to avoid arguments in the bathroom, kitchen, garage, near weapons, or in rooms without access to an outside door.)

I can tell the following people about the past violence and request they call the police if they hear suspicious noises coming from my home:

1. _____

2. _____

3. _____

I will use _____ as my code word with my children/family/friends so they can call for help.

Safety When Preparing to Leave

Victims sometimes need to leave the residence they share with the abusive partner. Abusers often explode when they believe that a victim is leaving the relationship. Leaving home must be done with a careful plan in order to increase safety. Following is a sample action plan:

If I have to leave my home, I will go

_____

_____

I can leave copies of important documents, an extra set of car and/or house keys, money, and extra clothes with

_____

_____

I will have important phone numbers accessible to my children and myself. The phone located nearest to my home is located at

_____

_____

I will check with the following people to see who would be able to let me stay with them:

1. _____

2. _____

3. _____

When I leave I will need to take:

- Identification for myself (driver's license or ID)
- Social security cards for all family members
- Birth certificates for all family members
- School and vaccination records for children
- Medications for all family members
- Divorce/custody papers
- Work permits/green card/passports
- Money/checkbook/ATM and credit cards/bank book
- Children's favorite toys/blankets
- Lease/rental agreement, mortgage payment book, house deed

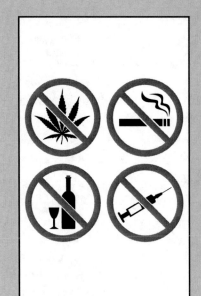

Chapter 9
Alcohol, Tobacco, and Drugs

Alcohol

The use and abuse of alcohol is a serious problem in U.S. society.

Statistics[117]

- Approximately 14 million Americans—7.4 percent of the population—meet the diagnostic criteria for alcohol abuse or alcoholism.
- More than one-half of American adults have a close family member who has or has had alcoholism.
- Approximately one in four children younger than 18 years old in the United States are exposed to alcohol abuse or alcohol dependence in the family.

Almost half of Americans aged 12 or older reported being current drinkers of alcohol in the 2001 survey (48.3 percent). This translates to an estimated 109 million people. The highest prevalence of both heavy drinking and binge-drinking in 2001 was for young adults aged 18 to 25, with the peak rate occurring at age 21.[118]

Alcoholism, also known as alcohol dependence, is a disease that includes four symptoms:

- Craving: A strong need, or compulsion, to drink.
- Loss of control: The inability to limit one's drinking on any given occasion.
- Physical dependence: Withdrawal symptoms, such as nausea, sweating, shakiness, and anxiety, occur when alcohol use is stopped after a period of heavy drinking.
- Tolerance: The need to drink greater amounts of alcohol in order to "get high."

Alcoholism and drug addiction is taking a toll on the American family. As a result, 8.3 million children in the United States, approximately 11 percent, live with at least one parent who is in need of treatment for alcohol or drug dependency. One in four children under the age of 18 are living in a home where alcoholism or alcohol abuse is a fact of daily life. Countless others are exposed to illegal drug use in their families.[119]

Children of addiction are at significantly greater risk for:

- Mental illness or emotional problems, such as depression or anxiety
- Physical health problems

- Learning problems, including difficulty with cognitive and verbal skills, conceptual reasoning, and abstract thinking
- Children whose parents abuse alcohol or drugs are almost three times more likely to be verbally, physically, or sexually abused and four times more likely than other children to be neglected.
- Developing alcoholism or other drug problems[120]

Brief History of Minimum Legal Drinking Age

The Eighteenth Amendment to the U.S. Constitution was passed in 1919 and was made effective in 1920. This started the period known as Prohibition. The Eighteenth Amendment declared that alcohol could not be manufactured, sold, imported, exported, or transported in the United States. In 1933, the Twenty-First Amendment to the Constitution was passed, which repealed the Eighteenth Amendment and made alcohol legal again. After Prohibition, nearly all states restricting youth access to alcohol designated 21 as the minimum legal drinking age (MLDA). Between 1970 and 1975, however, 29 states lowered the MLDA to 18, 19, or 20. These changes occurred when the minimum age for other activities, such as voting, also were being lowered. Scientists began studying the effects of the lowered MLDA, focusing particularly on the incidence of motor vehicle crashes, the leading cause of death among teenagers. Several studies in the 1970s found that motor vehicle crashes increased significantly among teens when the MLDA was lowered.[121]

What Is a Standard Drink?

- 12 oz. of beer or cooler
- 5 oz. of wine
- 1.5 oz. of spirits (hard liquor)

Blood Alcohol Concentration

The amount of alcohol in your body is commonly measured by the blood alcohol concentration (BAC). BAC is the amount of alcohol in the bloodstream. It is measured in percentages. For instance, having a BAC of 0.10 percent means that a person has 1 part alcohol per 1,000 parts blood in the body. BAC is estimated from breath ethanol content measured with a machine commonly referred to as a breathalyzer. BAC can be measured by breath, blood, or urine tests.

The legal intoxication level in most states is 0.08 percent BAC. But because alcohol depresses the central nervous system, causing slowed reactions, one's ability to drive is affected long before a BAC of 0.08 percent is reached.

In some states, drivers under 21 are considered legally impaired at lower levels (perhaps 0.02) as part of a zero-tolerance policy.

Factors Affecting BAC

- *How much* alcohol you drink.
- *How fast you drink.* The quicker you drink, the higher your peak BAC will be. The liver gets rid of alcohol at the average rate of one drink per hour (12 oz. beer, 5 oz. wine, 1 shot of distilled liquor). If a person drinks faster than this, the remainder will circulate in the bloodstream until the liver can get rid of it.
- *Weight.* Heavier people will be less affected by the same amount of alcohol than lighter people. They have more blood and water in their bodies in which to dilute the alcohol.
- *Food in the stomach.* When there is food in the stomach, alcohol is absorbed slower into the bloodstream. The BAC rises more rapidly in those who drink on an empty stomach, because there is no food in which to dilute the alcohol.

172

- *The type of alcohol you drink.* The stronger a drink is (the higher the alcohol concentration, distilled alcohol first, wine second, beer third), the more quickly it is absorbed. This partially explains why hard liquor has more of an apparent "kick" than wine or beer.
- *Type of mixer used.* Water and fruit juices mixed with alcohol slow the absorption process, whereas carbonated beverages will speed it up. Carbon dioxide speeds the alcohol through the stomach and intestine into the bloodstream, creating a rapid rise in BAC.
- *Temperature of the drink.* Warm alcohol is absorbed quicker than cold alcohol.
- *Drinking history/tolerance.* If there is a long history of drinking, increasing amounts of alcohol are needed to result in the physical and behavioral reactions formerly produced at lesser concentrations.
- *General state of emotional and mental health.* Many people seem more susceptible to the effects of alcohol when they are extremely fatigued, have recently been ill, or are under emotional stress and strain. The usual amount of alcohol may result in uncomfortable effects.
- *Other drugs.* Prescription, over-the-counter, illicit, and unrecognized drugs all have potential reactions with alcohol. One should be aware of the additive and synergistic effects when these drugs are mixed with alcohol.
- Males and females respond differently to the effects of alcohol.

Females Process Alcohol Differently than Males

1. *Less body water in women.* For a male and female of the same weight, females have less amount of water in their body. In addition, females tend to weigh less than men. With less of their body containing water and weighing less in general, the same amount of alcohol will be more intoxicating for a female.
2. *Alcohol metabolism.* Females burn up alcohol less rapidly than males. The enzyme (alcohol dehydrogenase) in the stomach that burns up (metabolizes) alcohol is 25 percent less active in females. That means higher levels of alcohol reach their blood and brain, producing greater intoxication.
3. *Hormone levels.* Changing hormonal levels at certain times during the menstrual cycle increase the level of alcohol in a female's body. A woman drinking the same amount of alcohol every day will have twice or more the level of alcohol in her blood during the middle of the menstrual cycle around the time of ovulation as she will at other times in her cycle.

Effects of Alcohol

- *Brain.* Alcohol is a "downer." It directly affects the brain cells. Unclear thinking, staggering, and slurred speech may result. Drinking a high concentration of alcohol in a short period of time can suppress the centers of the brain that control breathing, causing a person to pass out or even die.
- *Eyes.* Alcohol causes blurred vision.
- *Heart.* Alcohol can increase the workload of the heart. Irregular heartbeat and high blood pressure can result. At intoxicating doses, alcohol can decrease heart rate, lower blood pressure and respiration rate, and result in decreased reflex responses and slower reaction times.
- *Liver.* Alcohol can poison the liver. Prolonged use causes extensive damage and organ failure.
- *Stomach/Pancreas.* Alcohol irritates the digestive system. Vomiting and ulcers may result.
- *Kidneys.* Alcohol can stop the kidneys from maintaining a proper balance of body fluids and minerals.
- *Veins/Arteries.* Alcohol widens blood vessels, causing headaches and loss of body heat. It also lowers body temperature—this dilation of vessels actually causes heat loss from the extremities, which makes you more vulnerable to the cold. The vessels constrict in the first place to conserve heat, a defense the alcohol undoes.

- *Blood.* Alcohol reduces your body's ability to produce blood cells, resulting in anemia and/or infections.
- *Muscles.* Alcohol can cause muscle weakness, including weakness of the heart muscle.

Path of Alcohol in the Body

1. *Mouth:* alcohol enters the body.
2. *Stomach:* some alcohol gets into the bloodstream in the stomach, but most goes on to the small intestine.
3. *Small intestine:* alcohol enters the bloodstream through the walls of the small intestine.
4. *Heart:* pumps alcohol throughout the body.
5. *Brain:* alcohol reaches the brain.
6. *Liver:* alcohol is oxidized by the liver at a rate of about 0.5 oz. per hour. Alcohol is converted into water, carbon dioxide, and energy.

The Toll of Drinking[122]

- The Centers for Disease Control and Prevention (CDC) estimates that 4,554 underage deaths each year are due to excessive alcohol use.
- Alcohol use plays a substantial role in all three leading causes of death among youth—unintentional injuries (including motor vehicle fatalities and drowning), suicides, and homicides.
- Among young people, binge drinkers and heavy drinkers are more than twice as likely as non-drinkers to report having attempted to injure themselves or having contemplated or attempted to commit suicide.
- Three teens are killed each day when they drink alcohol and drive. At least six more die every day from other alcohol-related causes.
- According to the National Highway Traffic Safety Administration, 6,002 young people ages 16 to 20 died in motor vehicle crashes in 2003. Alcohol was involved in 38 percent of these deaths.
- It is estimated that teenage girls who binge-drink are up to 63 percent more likely to become teen mothers.
- There is growing evidence to suggest that alcohol use prior to age 21 impairs crucial aspects of youthful brain development.

Results of Chronic Alcohol Abuse

- Cirrhosis of the liver
- Damage the frontal lobes of the brain
- Overall reduction in brain size and increase in the size of the ventricles (fluid-filled cavities)
- Alcoholism (addiction to alcohol) and tolerance to the effects of alcohol and variety of health problems
- Vitamin deficiency—because the digestion system of alcoholics is unable to absorb vitamin B_1 (thiamine), a syndrome known as *Wernicke's encephalopathy* may develop. This syndrome is characterized by impaired memory, confusion, and lack of coordination.
- Further deficiencies of thiamine can lead to *Korsakoff's syndrome*. This disorder is characterized by amnesia, apathy, and disorientation.

Fetal Alcohol Syndrome (FAS)

Compared to normal babies, babies born with FAS have:

- Smaller heads and brains
- Some degree of mental retardation
- Poor coordination
- Hyperactivity
- Abnormal facial features
- Lower IQ

Positive Effects of Alcohol

- In light drinkers, there is less heart disease than in nondrinkers. However, there's more cancer.
- Recommendation: one drink a day for women and two drinks a day for men.
- Wine has the healthiest effects.

Binge Drinking

Binge drinking is defined as drinking five or more drinks on the same occasion (i.e., within a few hours) on at least 1 day in the past 30 days.

Consequences

Drinking by college students aged 18 to 24 contributes to an estimated 1,700 student deaths, 599,000 injuries, and 97,000 cases of sexual assault or date rape each year.[123]

What Happens to Your Body When You Get Alcohol Poisoning?

- Alcohol depresses nerves that control involuntary actions such as breathing and the gag reflex (which prevents choking). A fatal dose of alcohol will eventually stop these functions. Alcohol has a built-in safety feature: We either vomit or pass out before we have a chance to kill ourselves. The trick is not to do the two things simultaneously; otherwise you risk choking on your own vomit.
- When people pass out, their bodies continue to absorb alcohol. The amount of alcohol in the blood can reach dangerous levels, and they can die in their sleep. Continue to check on someone who has gone to sleep drunk. Do not leave that person alone.
- A person's BAC can continue to rise even while he or she is passed out. Even after a person stops drinking, alcohol in the stomach and intestine continues to enter the bloodstream and circulate throughout the body. It is dangerous to assume the person will be fine by sleeping it off.

Critical Signs for Alcohol Poisoning

- Mental confusion, stupor, coma, or person cannot be roused
- Vomiting
- Seizures
- Slow breathing (fewer than eight breaths per minute)
- Irregular breathing (10 seconds or more between breaths)
- Hypothermia (low body temperature), bluish skin color, paleness

What Should I Do If I Suspect Someone Has Alcohol Poisoning?

- Know the danger signals.
- Do not wait for all symptoms to be present.
- Be aware that a person who has passed out may die.
- If there is any suspicion of an alcohol overdose, call 911 for help. Don't try to guess the level of drunkenness.

What Can Happen to Someone with Alcohol Poisoning That Goes Untreated?

- Victim may choke on his or her own vomit.
- Breathing may slow, become irregular, or stop.
- Heart may beat irregularly or stop.
- Hypothermia (low body temperature) may result.
- Hypoglycemia (too little blood sugar) may lead to seizures.
- Untreated severe dehydration from vomiting can cause seizures, permanent brain damage, or death.
- Even if the victim lives, an alcohol overdose can lead to irreversible brain damage.

Reasons to Quit Binge Drinking

- To reduce chances of dying in a car crash
- To decrease the chance of falls or other injuries
- To do better in school
- To decrease chances of being date raped
- To prevent blackouts
- To decrease the chance of contracting STDs
- To save money
- To feel better
- To have more energy
- To be nicer to my friends
- To reduce my weight
- To reduce the number of headaches
- To reduce stomach pain
- To reduce risk of developing an addiction to alcohol
- To decrease chance of developing medical problems related to drinking

Advertising and Youth

- A study published in January 2006 concludes that greater exposure to alcohol advertising contributes to an increase in drinking among underage youth. Specifically, for each additional ad a young person saw above the average for youth, he or she was 1 percent more likely to drink. For each additional dollar spent per capita on alcohol advertising in a local market, young people drank 3 percent more.[124]
- Young people view approximately 20,000 commercials each year, of which nearly 2,000 are for beer and wine. For every "just say no" or "know when to say when" public service announcement, teens will view 25 to 50 beer and wine commercials.[125]

- In 2000, brewers spent more than $770 million on television ads and $15 million more on radio. Since dropping its own TV ad ban in 1996, liquor-industry expenditures on broadcast commercials (primarily on cable TV) skyrocketed from $3.5 million to more than $25 million in 2000.[126]
- Diageo, maker of Smirnoff Vodka, Captain Morgan's Rum, and Cuervo Tequila, has announced plans to spend as much as $1 billion on television liquor ads over the next five years.[127]

Alcohol Marketing and the African American Community[128]

- Alcohol is the drug most widely used by African American youth.[129]
- Although African American youth drink less than other youth, there is evidence from public health research that, as they age, African Americans suffer more from alcohol-related diseases than other groups in the population.[130]
- Battles over the heavy marketing to the African American community of malt liquor, a stronger-than-average beer, resulted in the banning of one new brand, PowerMaster, and fines against the makers of another, St. Ides Malt Liquor, by the states of New York and Oregon, for advertising practices that allegedly targeted youth and glamorized gang activity.
- References to alcohol were more frequent in rap (47 percent of songs had alcohol references) than other genres such as country-western (13 percent), top 40 (12 percent), alternative rock (10 percent), and heavy metal (4 percent); and 48 percent of these rap songs had product placements or mentions of specific alcohol brand names.

Alcohol and Medication Effects

1. *Antibiotics*—Alcohol decreases effects of certain antibiotics.
2. *Anticoagulants (Coumadin)*—Alcohol can lead to risk of life-threatening hemorrhages.
3. *Antidepressants and antipsychotics*—Alcohol increases the sedative effect of some, impairing mental skills required for driving. A chemical called tyramine, found in some beers and wine, interacts with some antidepressants, such as monoamine oxidase inhibitors, to produce a dangerous rise in blood pressure.
4. *Aspirin* (nonnarcotic pain relievers)—Some of these drugs cause stomach bleeding and inhibit blood from clotting; alcohol can exacerbate these effects.
5. *Acetaminophen*—liver damage.
6. *Antihistamines*—Alcohol may intensify the sedation.
7. *Narcotic pain relievers*—The combination of opiates and alcohol enhances the sedative effect of both substances, increasing the risk of death from overdose.
8. *Sedatives and hypnotics* (sleeping pills) cause severe drowsiness in the presence of alcohol.
9. *Antidiabetic medication*—Alcohol causes blood sugar fluctuations.
10. *Antiseizure medications*—Alcohol increases the risk of drug-related side effects.
11. *Antiulcer medications* increase the availability of a low dose of alcohol under some circumstances.
12. *Cardiovascular medications*—Alcohol causes dizziness, fainting.

Withdrawal

People who drink all the time build up a tolerance to alcohol. Symptoms are:

- Tremors
- Irritability

- Anxiety
- Heightened sensitivity to light, noise, and pain
- Hallucinations
- Convulsions

Hangovers

- *Coffee or a cold shower will not sober you up if you're drunk.*
- Only time can make you sober. It takes approximately two hours for each ounce of alcohol to work its way out of your bloodstream.
- Drink plenty of water.
- Do not take Tylenol or other medications.

How Can You Tell If a Friend Has a Drinking Problem?

If your friend has one or more of the following warning signs, he or she may have a problem with alcohol:

- Getting drunk on a regular basis
- Lying about how much alcohol he or she is using
- Believing that alcohol is necessary to have fun
- Having frequent hangovers
- Feeling run-down, depressed, or even suicidal
- Having "blackouts"—forgetting what he or she did while drinking

What Can You Do to Help Someone Who Has a Drinking Problem?

For information and referrals, call the National Clearinghouse for Alcohol and Drug Information at 1-800-729-6686.

Cigarettes

Smoking is the most preventable cause of premature death in our society.

Who Smokes?[131]

According to the Centers for Disease Control and Prevention (CDC), 44.5 million U.S. adults were current smokers in 2004 (the most recent year for which numbers are available). This is 20.9 percent of all adults (23.4 percent of men, 18.5 percent of women)—more than one out of five people.

When broken down by race/ethnicity, the numbers for 2004 are as follows:

American Indians/Alaska Natives	33.4 percent
Whites	22.2 percent
African Americans	20.2 percent
Hispanics	15.0 percent
Asian Americans	11.3 percent

Health Effects of Smoking

- About half of all Americans who continue to smoke will die because of the habit.
- Nearly one of every five deaths is related to smoking. Cigarettes kill more Americans than alcohol, car accidents, suicide, AIDS, homicide, and illegal drugs combined.
- Smoking is the number-one preventable cause of death.
- About 87 percent of lung cancer deaths are caused by smoking.

Diseases Caused by Long-Term Smoking

- Cancer of the lung, mouth, nose, voice box, lip, tongue, nasal sinus, esophagus, throat, pancreas, bone marrow (myeloid leukaemia), kidney, cervix, liver, bladder, and stomach
- Lung diseases such as chronic obstructive pulmonary disease, which includes chronic bronchitis and emphysema
- Coronary artery disease, heart disease, heart attack, and stroke
- Ulcers of the digestive system
- Osteoporosis and hip fracture
- Poor blood circulation in feet and hands, which can lead to pain and, in severe cases, gangrene and amputation

The Female Body

When calling attention to public health problems, we must not misuse the word 'epidemic.' But there is no better word to describe the 600-percent increase since 1950 in women's death rates for lung cancer, a disease primarily caused by cigarette smoking. Clearly, smoking-related disease among women is a full-blown epidemic.

—David Satcher, MD, PhD

- The most recent CDC survey (from 2004) showed that about one in five American women (19 percent) smoked cigarettes. The highest rates were seen among American Indian and Alaska Native women (29 percent), followed by white (20 percent), African American (17 percent), Hispanic (11 percent), and Asian women (5 percent). The less education a woman has, the more likely she is to smoke.[132]
- Women who smoke greatly increase their risk of heart disease (the leading killer among women) and stroke.
- Some studies suggest that smoking cigarettes dramatically increases the risk of heart disease among younger women who are also taking birth control pills.

The specific effects of tobacco smoke on the female body include:

- reduced fertility.
- menstrual cycle irregularities or absence of menstruation.
- menopause reached one or two years earlier.
- increased risk of cancer of the cervix.
- greatly increased risk of stroke and heart attack if the smoker is over age 35 years and taking a oral contraceptive pill.

Birth control and smoking increases risk of:

- blood clots.
- strokes.
- heart disease.

The Male Body

The specific effects of tobacco smoke on the male body include:

- lower sperm count.
- higher percentage of deformed sperm.
- reduced sperm mobility.
- changed levels of male sex hormones.
- impotence, which may be due to the effects of smoking on blood flow and damage to the blood vessels of the penis.

The Effects of Maternal Smoking

- Increased risk of miscarriage, stillbirth, and premature birth
- Low birth weight, which may have a lasting effect on the growth and development of children. Low birth weight is associated with an increased risk for early puberty, and in adulthood an increased risk for heart disease, stroke, high blood pressure, and diabetes.
- Increased risk of cleft palate and cleft lip
- Paternal smoking can also harm the fetus if the nonsmoking mother is exposed to passive smoking.
- If the mother continues to smoke during her baby's first year of life, the child has an increased risk of ear infections, respiratory illnesses such as pneumonia, croup and bronchitis, sudden infant death syndrome (SIDS), and meningococcal disease.

Ingredients in Tobacco

Cigarettes, cigars, and smokeless and pipe tobacco consist of dried tobacco leaves, as well as ingredients added for flavor and other properties. More than 4,000 individual compounds have been identified in tobacco and tobacco smoke. Among these are more than 60 compounds that are known carcinogens (cancer-causing agents).

Some of the compounds found in tobacco smoke include:

- Tar (burning of tobacco)
- Carbon monoxide
- Cyanide
- Benzene
- Formaldehyde
- Methanol (wood alcohol)
- Acetylene (the fuel used in welding torches)
- Ammonia

How Nicotine Affects the Body

Nicotine is highly addictive. It is both a stimulant and a sedative to the central nervous system. The ingestion of nicotine results in almost immediate pleasure because it causes a discharge of epinephrine from the adrenal cortex. This stimulates the central nervous system and other endocrine glands, which causes a sudden release of glucose. Stimulation is then followed by depression and fatigue, leading the abuser to seek more nicotine. Nicotine is absorbed readily from tobacco smoke in the lungs, and it does not matter whether the tobacco smoke is from cigarettes, cigars, or pipes.

Nicotine is a drug found naturally in tobacco. It is highly addictive, as addictive as heroin and cocaine. The body becomes physically and psychologically dependent on nicotine.

Nicotine also is absorbed readily when tobacco is chewed. With regular use of tobacco, levels of nicotine accumulate in the body during the day and persist overnight. Thus, daily smokers or chewers are exposed to the effects of nicotine for 24 hours each day. Nicotine taken in by cigarette or cigar smoking takes only seconds to reach the brain but has a direct effect on the body for up to 30 minutes.

Research has shown that stress and anxiety affect nicotine tolerance and dependence. Stress hormones reduces the effects of nicotine; therefore, more nicotine must be consumed to achieve the same effect. This increases tolerance to nicotine and leads to increased dependence.

Addiction to nicotine results in withdrawal symptoms when a person tries to stop smoking. For example, a study found that when chronic smokers were deprived of cigarettes for 24 hours, they had increased anger, hostility, and aggression, and loss of social cooperation. Persons suffering from withdrawal also take longer to regain emotional equilibrium following stress. During periods of abstinence and/or craving, smokers have shown impairment across a wide range of psychomotor and cognitive functions, such as language comprehension.[133]

Tobacco companies are required by law to report nicotine levels in cigarettes to the Federal Trade Commission (FTC) but in most states are not required to show the amount of nicotine on the cigarette brand labeling. The actual amount of nicotine available to the smoker in a given brand of cigarettes may be different from the level reported to the FTC. In one regular cigarette, the amount of nicotine ranges between about 1 mg and 2 mg.[134]

Although 70 percent of smokers want to quit and 35 percent attempt to quit each year, fewer than 5 percent succeed. The low rate of successful quitting and the high rate of relapse are due to the effects of nicotine addiction.[135]

 Research has found that even smoking as few as one to four cigarettes a day can have serious health consequences, including an increased risk of heart disease and a higher risk of dying at an earlier age.

Secondhand Smoke

Secondhand smoke, also known as environmental tobacco smoke (ETS) or passive smoke, is a mixture of two forms of smoke from burning tobacco products:

- *Sidestream smoke:* smoke that comes from the end of a lighted cigarette, pipe, or cigar.
- *Mainstream smoke:* smoke that is exhaled by a smoker.

Secondhand smoke is classified as a "known human carcinogen." Secondhand tobacco smoke contains over 4,000 chemical compounds. Secondhand smoke can be harmful in many ways.

In the United States alone, secondhand smoke is responsible for:[136]

- an estimated 35,000 to 40,000 deaths from heart disease in people who are not current smokers.
- about 3,000 lung cancer deaths in nonsmoking adults.
- other respiratory problems in nonsmokers, including coughing, phlegm, chest discomfort, and reduced lung function.

- 150,000 to 300,000 lower respiratory tract infections (such as pneumonia and bronchitis) in children younger than 18 months of age, which result in 7,500 to 15,000 hospitalizations.
- increases in the number and severity of asthma attacks from about 200,000 to 1 million asthmatic children.
- increases in the risk of sudden infant death syndrome (SIDS) and middle ear infections in young children.
- low birth weight in babies whose mothers are exposed to ETS.

Third-hand Smoke

Doctors from Mass General Hospital for Children in Boston coined the term "third-hand smoke" to describe chemicals from the cigarettes by-products that cling to smokers' hair and clothing as well as to household fabrics, carpets, and surfaces, even after secondhand smoke has cleared.

This third-hand smoke is NOT cleared, even if you open a window or turn on a fan, and this poses a huge threat to children especially. Third-hand smoke is an invisible, cancer-causing toxic brew of gases and particles. This residue includes heavy metals and even radioactive materials that young children can get on their hands and ingest, especially if they're crawling or playing on the floor.

Spit (Smokeless Tobacco)

- Cancer of the mouth and pharynx
- Leukoplakia (white sores in the mouth that can lead to cancer)
- Gum recession, or peeling back of gums
- Bone loss around the teeth
- Abrasion of teeth
- Bad breath

Clove cigarettes, also called kreteks, are imported mainly from Indonesia and contain 60 to 70 percent tobacco and 30 to 40 percent ground cloves, clove oil, and other additives. The chemicals in cloves have been implicated in cases of asthma and other lung diseases.

Bidis are flavored cigarettes imported mainly from India. They are hand-rolled in an unprocessed tobacco leaf and tied with strings on the ends. Their popularity has grown in recent years in part because they come in a variety of candy-like flavors such as strawberry, vanilla, and grape, they are usually less expensive than regular cigarettes, and they often give the smoker an immediate buzz. They have higher levels of nicotine (the addictive chemical in tobacco) and other harmful substances such as tar and carbon monoxide. And because they are thinner than regular cigarettes, they require about three times as many puffs per cigarette. They are also unfiltered.

Most *cigars* have as much nicotine as several cigarettes. When cigar smokers inhale, nicotine is absorbed as rapidly as it is with cigarettes. For those who do not inhale, it is absorbed more slowly through the lining of the mouth. Smoking cigars causes cancers of the lung, oral cavity (lip, tongue, mouth, throat), larynx (voice box), esophagus, and probably cancers of the bladder and pancreas. Cigar smokers have a greater risk of dying from cancer of the oral cavity, larynx, or esophagus compared with nonsmokers.

Hookah smoking, which started in the Middle East, involves burning flavored tobacco in a water pipe and inhaling the smoke through a long hose. It has recently become popular among young people, especially around college campuses. It is marketed as being a safe alternative to cigarettes because the percent of tobacco in the product smoked is low. *This claim for safety is not true.* The water does not filter out many of the toxins, and hookah smoke contains varying amounts of nicotine, carbon monoxide, and other hazardous substances. Several types of cancer, as well as other health effects, have been linked to hookah smoking.

Are Menthol Cigarettes Safer than Other Brands?

Menthol cigarettes are not safer than other brands and may even be more dangerous. Menthol cigarettes produce a cool sensation in the throat when smoke is inhaled. People who smoke menthol cigarettes can inhale deeper and hold the smoke inside longer than smokers of nonmenthol cigarettes. About one-fourth of all cigarettes sold in the United States are flavored with menthol, and these cigarettes are especially popular among African American smokers.

Benefits of Quitting Smoking

In September 1990, the U.S. Surgeon General outlined the benefits of smoking cessation:[137]

- Smoking cessation has major and immediate health benefits for men and women of all ages. Benefits apply to persons with and without smoking-related disease.
- Former smokers live longer than continuing smokers. For example, persons who quit smoking before age 50 have one-half the risk of dying in the next 15 years compared with continuing smokers.
- Smoking cessation decreases the risk of lung cancer, other cancers, heart attack, stroke, and chronic lung disease.
- Women who stop smoking before pregnancy or during the first three to four months of pregnancy reduce their risk of having a low-birth-weight baby to that of women who never smoked.
- The health benefits of smoking cessation far exceed any risks from the average 5-pound (2.3-kg) weight gain or any adverse psychological effects that may follow quitting.
- The risk of having lung cancer and other smoking-related cancers is related to total lifetime exposure to cigarette smoke, as measured by the number of cigarettes smoked each day, the age at which smoking began, and the number of years a person has smoked.
- People who stop smoking at younger ages experience the greatest health benefits from quitting. Those who quit in their 30s may avoid most of the risk due to tobacco use. However, even smokers who quit after age 50 substantially reduce their risk of dying early. The argument that it is too late to quit smoking because the damage is already done is not true.

Quitting[138]

After 20 minutes: Your blood pressure drops to a level close to that before the last cigarette. The temperature of your hands and feet increases to normal.

After 8 hours: The carbon monoxide level in your blood drops to normal.

After 24 hours: Your chance of a heart attack decreases.

Within 3 months: Your circulation improves and your lung function increases up to 30 percent.

In 1 to 9 months: Coughing, sinus congestion, fatigue, and shortness of breath decrease; cilia (tiny hair-like structures that move mucus out of the lungs) regain normal function in the lungs, increasing the ability to handle mucus, clean the lungs, and reduce infection.

After 1 year: The excess risk of coronary heart disease is half that of a smoker's.

After 5 years: Stroke risk is reduced to that of a nonsmoker.

After 10 years: The lung cancer death rate is about half that of a continuing smoker's. The risk of cancer of the mouth, throat, esophagus, bladder, kidney, and pancreas decreases.

After 15 years: The risk of coronary heart disease is that of a nonsmoker's.

Cost of Smoking

How much do you pay for a pack of cigarettes? _____

How many cigarettes are you smoking each day? _____

Cost per day: _____

Cost per week: _____

Cost per month: _____

Cost per year: _____

Total cost to date: _____

What else could I have done with this money?

_____

_____

_____

_____

Drug Addiction

Why do college students use drugs?

_____

_____

_____

_____

Reasons for Drug Use

- Deal with stress
- Experimentation
- Pleasure/boredom
- Peer pressure
- Self-discovery
- Social interaction
- Rebelliousness

Addiction is characterized by compulsive drug craving, seeking, and use that persists even in the face of negative consequences.

All addicting drugs act on a single aspect of the brain: dopamine. Dopamine allows us to experience pleasure. Love, sex, food, movies, alcohol, and drugs all release chemicals in our brain that we feel as pleasure.

Our Brains Get Accustomed to Alcohol and Drugs

Drugs can cause such intense pleasure that we can stop wanting to do anything else but take drugs. Our brains change and get accustomed to having drugs. They stop reacting as strongly to the substance so we need to take more and more. The disease of addiction occurs as permanent changes in our brain develop from the repeated exposure to alcohol or addicting drugs.

Dependency Factors

- Genetic factors inherited from our parents
- Our childhood experiences (both with our family and peer group)
- Our current peer group and life situation
- The level of addictive and risk potential of the drugs we use

Common Dependency Defenses

- *Denial:* Refusing to admit or acknowledge that our drinking or using has become a problem. (I can quit any time I want to. My using isn't that bad.)
- *Isolation:* Removing ourselves from the company of family and friends for the purpose of maintaining a chemical habit.
- *Rationalization:* Giving reasons to explain why we drink or use. (I drink because I hate my job.)
- *Blaming:* Transferring responsibility for our behavior to other people. (I wouldn't drink if my spouse treated me right.)
- *Projection:* Rejecting our own feelings by ascribing them to someone else. (Why is that stupid idiot being so hostile?)
- *Minimizing:* Refusing to admit the magnitude of the amount used. (I only have a couple of drinks. It's not a problem.)

Diagnostic and Statistical Manual—IV (DSM-IV)[139]

The DSM-IV defines dependency as a maladaptive pattern of substance use leading to clinically significant impairment or distress as manifested by three (or more) of the following, occurring at any time in the same 12-month period:

- Substance is often taken in larger amounts or over longer period than intended.
- Persistent desire or unsuccessful efforts to cut down or control substance use.
- A great deal of time is spent in activities necessary to obtain the substance (e.g., visiting multiple doctors or driving long distances), use the substance (e.g., chain smoking), or recover from its effects.
- Important social, occupational, or recreational activities given up or reduced because of substance abuse.
- Continued substance use despite knowledge of having a persistent or recurrent psychological or physical problem that is caused or exacerbated by use of the substance.

- Tolerance, as defined by either:
    1. Pharmacological tolerance—need for real amounts of the substance in order to achieve intoxication or desired effect.
    2. Behavioral tolerance—an individual learns to adjust to the presence of drugs.
    3. Cross-tolerance—tolerance to a particular drug results in tolerance to chemically similar drugs.
    4. Reverse tolerance—markedly diminished effect with continued use of the same amount.
- Withdrawal, as manifested by either characteristic withdrawal syndrome for the substance, or the same (or closely related) substance is taken to relieve or avoid withdrawal symptoms.

Drug Interactions

- *Additive*—the cumulative effects of two or more substances added together.
- *Antagonistic*—drugs that negate each other's effects.
- *Synergism*—combined effects of two drugs are greater than if they were simply added together.

Examples:

- Alcohol and marijuana intensify each other's effects.
- Alcohol and tranquilizers → coma.
- Alcohol and antihistamines → deep sleep.
- Birth control and antibiotics → cancel the potency of the pill.
- Marijuana and cocaine → deadly heart rate and blood pressure.

In contrast to prescription drugs, illegal drugs are not manufactured in controlled environments under strict standards of quality. You never know what quality and quantity you are really getting, or with what cheaper poison an unscrupulous dealer may have diluted the drug.

Some of the side effects of illegal drugs could actually limit your ability to have the "good time" you might have thought the drug was going to provide. The side effects multiply, compound, and can cause permanent damage the more frequently you take the drugs.

Side Effects

- Confusion
- Anxiety
- Paranoia
- Panic attacks
- Nausea
- Shaking
- Headache
- Schizophrenic and psychotic behavior
- Hostile and aggressive behavior
- Violence, often for no apparent reason
- Periods of severe mental and emotional disturbance, and possible permanent mental illness
- Potentially permanent damage to brain, liver, kidneys, and heart

Most Dangerous Over-the-Counter Drugs

- Aspirin
- NSAIDs
- Acetaminophen
- Nasal sprays
- Laxatives
- Eye drops
- Cough syrup

Marijuana

Marijuana is the most commonly used illicit drug. Marijuana is a green, brown, or gray mixture of dried, shredded leaves, stems, seeds, and flowers of the hemp plant. All forms of marijuana are mind-altering. They all contain THC (delta-9-tetrahydrocannabinol), the main active chemical in marijuana. They also contain more than 400 other chemicals. Marijuana's effects on the user depend on its strength or potency, which is related to the amount of THC it contains. The THC content of marijuana has been increasing since the 1970s.[140]

■ *You cannot drive a vehicle for four to six hours after one marijuana cigarette.*

Short-Term Effects

Short-term effects of marijuana use include euphoria, slowed thinking and reaction time, confusion, impaired balance and coordination, increased heart rate and BP, increased anxiety and panic attacks, lowered fertility, and increased suicidal and schizophrenic thoughts.

Long-Term Effects[141]

Long-term effects of marijuana use include cough, frequent respiratory infections, impaired memory and learning, increased heart rate, anxiety, panic attacks, tolerance, addiction, heart disease, and cancer.

Effects of Marijuana on the Brain

Researchers have found that THC changes the way in which sensory information gets into and is processed by the hippocampus. The hippocampus is a component of the brain's limbic system that is crucial for learning, memory, and the integration of sensory experiences with emotions and motivations. Neurons in the information processing system of the hippocampus and the activity of the nerve fibers in this region are suppressed by THC. In addition, researchers have discovered that learned behaviors, which depend on the hippocampus, also deteriorate via this mechanism.

Recent research findings also indicate that long-term use of marijuana produces changes in the brain similar to those seen after long-term use of other major abused drugs.

Effects on the Lungs

Someone who smokes marijuana regularly may have many of the same respiratory problems as tobacco smokers. These individuals may have daily cough and phlegm, symptoms of chronic bronchitis, and more frequent chest colds. Continuing to smoke marijuana can lead to abnormal functioning of lung tissue injured or destroyed by marijuana smoke.

Regardless of the THC content, the amount of tar inhaled by marijuana smokers and the level of carbon monoxide absorbed are three to five times greater than among tobacco smokers. This may be due to the marijuana users' inhaling more deeply and holding the smoke in the lungs and because marijuana smoke is unfiltered. Benzopyrene (a carcinogen) is 70 percent higher in marijuana than tobacco.

Effects on Heart Rate and Blood Pressure

A marijuana user's heart rate can increase when using marijuana alone. Risk of heart attack triples within one hour of smoking one marijuana cigarette. Approximately 1 marijuana cigarette = 4 cigarettes; and has 50 percent more tar than tobacco smoke.

Effects of Heavy Marijuana Use on Learning and Social Behavior

A study of college students has shown that critical skills related to attention, memory, and learning are impaired among people who use marijuana heavily, even after discontinuing its use for at least 24 hours. These findings suggest that the greater impairment among heavy users is likely due to an alteration of brain activity produced by marijuana.

Longitudinal research on marijuana use among young people below college age indicates those who used marijuana have lower achievement than the nonusers, more acceptance of deviant behavior, more delinquent behavior and aggression, greater rebelliousness, poorer relationships with parents, and more associations with drug-using friends. Amotivational syndrome, or chronic apathy, is also a result.

Research also shows more anger and more regressive behavior (thumb sucking, temper tantrums) in toddlers whose parents use marijuana than among the toddlers of nonusing parents.

Effects on Pregnancy

Some studies have found that babies born to mothers who used marijuana during pregnancy were smaller than those born to mothers who did not use the drug. In general, smaller babies are more likely to develop health problems.

A nursing mother who uses marijuana passes some of the THC to the baby in her breastmilk. Research indicates that the use of marijuana by a mother during the first month of breastfeeding can impair the infant's motor development (control of muscle movement). Other studies confirm babies born with neurological defects and association to a rare childhood leukemia.

Addictive Potential

A drug is addicting if it causes compulsive, often uncontrollable drug craving, seeking, and use, even in the face of negative health and social consequences. Animal studies suggest marijuana causes physical dependence, and some people report withdrawal symptoms.

Withdrawal Symptoms

Symptoms of marijuana withdrawal include cravings, insomnia, restlessness, lower appetite, aggression, and mood swings.

Club Drugs

The term "club drugs" refers to a wide variety of drugs being used by young people at dance clubs, bars, and all-night dance parties ("trances" or "raves"). Because many of these drugs are colorless, tasteless, and odorless, they can be secretly added to beverages by individuals who want to intoxicate or sedate others.

Short-Term Effects

- Stimulation
- Loss of inhibition
- Headache

- Nausea or vomiting
- Slurred speech
- Loss of motor coordination
- Wheezing

Long-Term Effects

- Unconsciousness
- Cramps
- Weight loss
- Muscle weakness
- Depression
- Memory impairment
- Damage to cardiovascular and nervous systems
- Sudden death

Widely Used Club Drugs[142]

Ecstasy[143]

Also known as MDMA (methylenedioxymethamphetamine), Ecstasy is a stimulant that combines the effects of amphetamines and hallucinogens. Street names for MDMA include Ecstasy, Adam, XTC, hug, beans, and love drug. Ecstasy is known to cause brain damage. MDMA also is neurotoxic, and depletes serotonin from the brain.

Side Effects

- Increased heart rate, blood pressure, and body temperature
- Nausea and sweating
- Convulsions
- Hallucinations
- Paranoia
- Severe depression
- Breathing problems

Life-Threatening Effects

- High doses can cause a sharp increase in body temperature (malignant hyperthermia), leading to muscle breakdown and kidney and cardiovascular system failure.
- Can cause hyponatremia and swelling of the brain and overstimulation of the nervous system.

Rohypnol

Known as the "date rape drug," Rohypnol is a central nervous system depressant that produces sedative-hypnotic effects, muscle relaxation, and amnesia. Rohypnol has been a concern for the last few years because of its abuse as a date rape drug. People may unknowingly be given the drug, which, when mixed with alcohol, can incapacitate victims and prevent them from resisting sexual assault. Also, Rohypnol can be lethal when mixed with alcohol and/or other depressants.

Rohypnol produces sedative-hypnotic effects including muscle relaxation and amnesia; it can also produce dependence. Rohypnol is not approved for use in the United States and its importation is banned. Illicit use of Rohypnol began in Europe in the 1970s and started appearing in the United

States in the early 1990s, where it became known as "rophies," "roofies," "roach," "rope," and the "date rape" drug.

Another very similar drug is clonazepam, marketed in the United States as Klonopin and in Mexico as Rivotril. It is sometimes abused to enhance the effects of heroin and other opiates.[144]

Ketamine

A rapid-acting general anesthetic and hallucinogen, ketamine produces a wide range of feelings, from weightlessness to out-of-body or near-death experiences. Ketamine (ketamine hydrochloride) is a central nervous system depressant that produces a rapid-acting dissociative effect. It was developed in the 1970s as a medical anesthetic for both humans and animals. Ketamine is often mistaken for cocaine or crystal methamphetamine because of its similar appearance.

Also known as K, Special K, Vitamin K, Kit Kat, Keller, Super Acid, and Super C, ketamine is available in tablet, powder, and liquid form. So powerful is the drug that, when injected, there is a risk of losing motor control before the injection is completed. In powder form, the drug can be snorted or sprinkled on tobacco or marijuana and smoked. The effects of ketamine last from 1 to 6 hours, and it is usually 24 to 48 hours before the user feels completely "normal" again.

GHB (Gamma Hydroxybutyrate)[145]

Originally available over the counter in health food stores to aid bodybuilders, GHB and other synthetic steroids are also used for their euphoric effects. GHB is a central nervous system depressant once used by many bodybuilders and athletes. In the 1980s, GHB was widely available over the counter in health food stores, and bodybuilders used it to lose fat and build muscle. GHB has been given nicknames such as Grievous Bodily Harm, G, Liquid Ecstasy, and Georgia Home Boy.

In 1990, the FDA banned the use of GHB except under the supervision of a physician because of reports of severe side effects, including euphoric and sedative effects similar to the effects experienced after taking Rohypnol (the "date rape" drug.) Because it clears from the body relatively quickly, it is often difficult to detect when patients go to emergency rooms and other treatment facilities.

Amphetamines

Amphetamines refers to various nervous system stimulants. Originally given to World War II soldiers to combat fatigue, amphetamines are widely prescribed for weight control and suppression of appetite. Because amphetamines trigger the release of adrenalin, they produce energy and alertness, and the user feels "wired."

1. Methamphetamine

Methamphetamine is made easily in laboratories with relatively inexpensive over-the-counter ingredients. These factors combine to make methamphetamine a drug with high potential for widespread abuse.

Methamphetamine is commonly known as "speed," "meth," and "chalk." In its smoked form, it is often referred to as "ice," "crystal," "crank," and "glass." It is a white, odorless, bitter-tasting crystalline powder that easily dissolves in water or alcohol. It was used originally in nasal decongestants and bronchial inhalers. Methamphetamine's chemical structure is similar to that of amphetamine, but it has more pronounced effects on the central nervous system. Like amphetamine, it causes increased activity, decreased appetite, and a general sense of well-being. The effects of methamphetamine can last six to eight hours. After the initial "rush," there is typically a state of high agitation that in some individuals can lead to violent behavior.[146]

Methamphetamine releases high levels of the neurotransmitter dopamine, which stimulates brain cells, enhancing mood and body movement. It also appears to have a neurotoxic effect, damaging brain cells that contain dopamine and serotonin. Over time, methamphetamine appears to cause reduced levels of dopamine, which can result in symptoms like those of Parkinson's disease, a severe movement disorder.[147]

Short-Term Effects

- Increased heart rate, blood pressure, and metabolism
- Feelings of exhilaration
- Energy
- Increased mental alertness
- Aggression, violence, psychotic behavior
- Suicidal thoughts.

Long-Term Effects

- Memory loss
- Cardiac and neurological damage
- Impaired memory and learning
- Tolerance, addiction
- Respiratory problems
- Irregular heartbeat
- Extreme anorexia
- Hyperthermia and convulsions can result in death.
- Increased heart rate and blood pressure can cause irreversible damage to blood vessels in the brain, producing strokes.
- Its use can result in cardiovascular collapse and death.

    Withdrawal symptoms are very intense. The user crashes intensely and desperately craves the drug.

2. Ritalin and Adderall

The United States uses approximately 90 percent of the world's ritalin. Most recently, major civil suits have been brought against Novartis, the manufacturer of ritalin, for fraud in the overpromotion of ADHD and ritalin. Furthermore, their addiction and abuse potential is based on the capacity of these drugs to drastically and permanently change brain chemistry. Studies of amphetamine show that short-term clinical doses produce brain cell death. Similar studies of ritalin show long-lasting and sometimes permanent changes in the biochemistry of the brain.[148]

All stimulants impair growth not only by suppressing appetite but also by disrupting growth hormone production. This poses a threat to every organ of the body, including the brain, during the child's growth. The disruption of neurotransmitter systems adds to this threat.

These drugs also endanger the cardiovascular system and commonly produce many adverse mental effects, including depression.

Side Effects

- Suicidal thoughts
- Nervousness and insomnia
- Hypersensitivity
- Anorexia
- Nausea, dizziness
- Palpitations

- Headache
- Drowsiness
- Blood pressure and pulse changes, both up and down
- Tachycardia, angina, cardiac arrhythmia
- Abdominal pain
- Weight loss
- There have been rare reports of Tourette's syndrome.
- Toxic psychosis has been reported.[149]

Hallucinogens

Hallucinogens are drugs that cause hallucinations—profound distortions in a person's perceptions of reality. Under the influence of hallucinogens, people see images, hear sounds, and feel sensations that seem real but do not exist. Some hallucinogens also produce rapid, intense emotional swings.

Hallucinogens cause their effects by disrupting the interaction of nerve cells and the neurotransmitter serotonin. Distributed throughout the brain and spinal cord, the serotonin system is involved in the control of behavioral, perceptual, and regulatory systems, including mood, hunger, body temperature, sexual behavior, muscle control, and sensory perception.

Short-Term Effects

- Increased heart rate and blood pressure
- Impaired motor function
- Possible decrease in blood pressure and heart rate
- Panic, aggression, and violence

Long-Term Effects

- Memory loss
- Numbness
- Nausea/vomiting
- Loss of appetite
- Depression
  1. **LSD (lysergic acid diethylamide):** This hallucinogen produces unpredictable effects, depending on the amount taken, the surroundings in which the drug is used, and the user's personality, mood, and expectations. LSD is tasteless, odorless, and colorless, and can be taken in different ways (e.g., on a sugar cube or tablet or placed on a blotter and licked). Behavior effects lasts six to eight hours. Fear or panic may lead to a "bad trip." Flashbacks are sometimes experienced because the drug remains in the spinal fluid.
  2. **Peyote:** Used by Aztec Indians for religious rituals. Until 1990 it was legally used in the United States by Native Americans. It comes from a cactus, and is the psychoactive agent in mescaline. Peyote takes effect within 30–90 minutes and stays in the body for about 10 hours. Hallucinogenic effects last for about two hours. Tolerance for peyote forms quickly.
  3. **Psilocybin:** Also called magic mushrooms or "shrooms"; the hallucinations produced by psilocybin are both visual and auditory. Psilocybin can produce responses from uncontrolled laughter to depression. Hallucinogenic effects are experienced within 30 minutes and can last 3 to 8 hours.

4. **PCP** ("PeaCe Pill"): PCP is an anesthetic capable of producing hallucinations; it can be smoked or ingested. Absorption is rapid and effects are experienced quickly. Acute effects lasts four to six hours. One may be in a state of confusion for 8 to 24 hours. Sometimes marijuana is laced with PCP, called a "killer joint" or "sherms." High doses can lead to coma, death, and violent behavior.

Heroin[150]

Heroin is a highly addictive drug, and its use is a serious problem in America. Recent studies suggest a shift from injecting heroin to snorting or smoking because of increased purity and the misconception that these forms of use will not lead to addiction.

Heroin is processed from morphine, a naturally occurring substance extracted from the seedpod of the Asian poppy plant. Heroin usually appears as a white or brown powder. Street names for heroin include "smack," "H," "skag," and "junk." Other names may refer to types of heroin produced in a specific geographical area, such as "Mexican black tar."

Short-Term Effects

Heroin abuse is associated with serious health conditions, including fatal overdose, spontaneous abortion, collapsed veins, and infectious diseases, including HIV/AIDS and hepatitis. It's one of the most deadliest drugs due to risk of overdose.

Heroin is a depressant. The short-term effects of heroin abuse appear soon after a single dose and disappear in a few hours. After an injection of heroin, the user reports feeling a surge of euphoria ("rush") accompanied by a warm flushing of the skin, a dry mouth, and heavy extremities. Following this initial euphoria, the user goes "on the nod," an alternately wakeful and drowsy state. Mental functioning becomes clouded due to the depression of the central nervous system.

In addition to the effects of the drug itself, street heroin may have additives that do not readily dissolve and result in clogging the blood vessels that lead to the lungs, liver, kidneys, or brain. This can cause infection or even death of small patches of cells in vital organs.

Long-Term Effects[151]

With regular heroin use, tolerance develops. This means the abuser must use more heroin to achieve the same intensity or effect. As higher doses are used over time, physical dependence and addiction develop. Chronic users may develop collapsed veins, infection of the heart lining and valves, abscesses, cellulitis, liver disease, and HIV. Pulmonary complications, including various types of pneumonia, may result from the poor health condition of the abuser, as well as from heroin's depressing effects on respiration.

Withdrawal, which in regular abusers may occur as early as a few hours after the last administration, produces drug craving, restlessness, muscle and bone pain, insomnia, diarrhea and vomiting, cold flashes with goose bumps ("cold turkey"), kicking movements ("kicking the habit"), and other symptoms. Major withdrawal symptoms peak between 48 and 72 hours after the last dose and subside after about a week.

Cocaine[152]

Cocaine is a powerfully addictive stimulant that directly affects the brain. Pure cocaine was first extracted from the leaf of the coca bush, which grows primarily in Peru and Bolivia, in the mid-nineteenth century. In the early 1900s, it became the main stimulant drug used in most of the tonics/elixirs that were developed to treat a wide variety of illnesses. Today, cocaine is a Schedule II drug, meaning that it has high potential for abuse but can be administered by a doctor for legitimate medical uses, such as a local anesthetic for some eye, ear, and throat surgeries.

There are basically two chemical forms of cocaine: the hydrochloride salt and the "freebase." The hydrochloride salt, or powdered form of cocaine, dissolves in water and, when abused, can be taken intravenously (by vein) or intranasally (in the nose). *Freebase* refers to a compound that has not been neutralized by an acid to make the hydrochloride salt. The freebase form of cocaine is smokable. The high from snorting may last 15 to 30 minutes, and that from smoking may last 5 to 10 minutes.

Cocaine is generally sold on the street as a fine, white, crystalline powder, and is also known as "coke," "C," "snow," "flake," or "blow." Street dealers generally dilute it with such inert substances as cornstarch, talcum powder, and/or sugar, or with such active drugs as procaine (a chemically related local anesthetic) or with other stimulants such as amphetamines.

Short-Term Effects

- Increased heart rate, blood pressure, and metabolism
- Feelings of exhilaration
- Energy
- Increased mental alertness
- Increased body temperature

Long-Term Effects[153]

Long-term effects include rapid or irregular heart beat, reduced appetite; weight loss, heart failure, chest pain, respiratory failure, nausea, abdominal pain, strokes, seizures, headaches, and malnutrition.

High doses of cocaine and/or prolonged use can trigger paranoia. When addicted individuals stop using cocaine, they often become depressed. This also may lead to further cocaine use to alleviate depression. Prolonged cocaine snorting can result in ulceration of the mucous membrane of the nose and can damage the nasal septum enough to cause it to collapse. Cocaine-related deaths are often a result of cardiac arrest or seizures followed by respiratory arrest.

When people mix cocaine and alcohol consumption, they are compounding the danger each drug poses and unknowingly forming a complex chemical experiment within their bodies. The human liver combines cocaine and alcohol and manufactures a third substance, cocaethylene, which intensifies cocaine's euphoric effects, while possibly increasing the risk of sudden death.

Crack

Crack is the street name given to the freebase form of cocaine that has been processed from the powdered cocaine hydrochloride form to a smokable substance. The term *crack* refers to the crackling sound heard when the mixture is smoked. Crack cocaine is processed with ammonia or sodium bicarbonate (baking soda) and water, and heated to remove the hydrochloride.

Because crack is smoked, the user experiences a high in less than 10 seconds. This rather immediate and euphoric effect is one of the reasons that crack became enormously popular in the mid-1980s. Another reason is that crack is inexpensive both to produce and buy. Smoking crack cocaine can produce a particularly aggressive paranoid behavior in users.

Inhalants[154]

Inhalants are breathable chemical vapors that produce psychoactive (mind-altering) effects. Although people are exposed to volatile solvents and other inhalants in the home and in the workplace, many do not think of inhalable substances as drugs because most of them were never meant to be used in that way.

Young people are likely to abuse inhalants, in part because inhalants are readily available and inexpensive. Sometimes children unintentionally misuse inhalants that are found in household products.

Short-Term Effects

- Impaired physical coordination
- Facial flushing
- Mental confusion
- Hallucinations
- Asphyxia

Long-Term Effects

- Sudden Sniffing Death
- Blindness
- Fatal damage of liver and kidneys

How to Avoid Tempting Situations

In certain situations, especially if you are having a bad day, you will find that you are tempted to drink, smoke, or take drugs. It is important to figure out ahead of time how to make sure you will not drink when you are tempted. Here are some tips from other students about ways to cope without drinking when life gets you down.

- Think of something pleasant you can do for yourself or for a friend.
- Telephone a sober friend.
- Exercise: go for a walk, play a sport, or go to the gym.
- Take a hot bath or shower.
- Watch a light movie or read a book or magazine.
- Write your feelings down in a notebook.
- Listen to music.
- *Surround yourself with positive people.*

Treatment

Chemical dependency is a treatable condition. The first goal of treatment is abstinence. The chemically dependent person must stop using alcohol or drugs. This sometimes requires a period of medical detoxification.

Once alcohol and/or drug use is stopped, individuals may honestly feel that they have the desire and ability to remain sober. This period can last days, weeks, or months before cravings (the obsessive pressure to use) return. To reduce the risk of a relapse the person must address personal problems and life issues related to the chemical dependency.

Participation in various self-help programs such as **Alcoholics Anonymous** and **Narcotics Anonymous** can help break addictions.

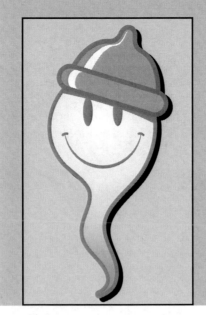

Chapter 10

Sexual Health

Sexual Health

Sexuality is a crucial aspect of human life and functioning. Many issues, both physical and mental, are interwoven together to form our sense of sexuality.

The Female

Each month the woman produces an egg from one of her two ovaries, which lie one on each side of the uterus (womb). The ovaries are glands that store the eggs in small sacs called follicles. Once the egg is released, fine hairs at the end of one of the fallopian tubes pick it up and bring it into the fallopian tube.

The egg then travels down the fallopian tube into the uterus. If it has been fertilized, the egg implants itself into the lining of the uterus (the endometrium). During each cycle the endometrium thickens, becoming ready to receive a fertilized egg. If there is no fertilized egg, the endometrium breaks down and is shed from the body at menstruation.

The Male

When the male ejaculates (which is when semen leaves a man's penis), between 0.05 and 0.2 fluid ounces (1.5 to 6.0 milliliters) of semen is deposited into the vagina. Between 75 and 900 million sperm are in this small amount of semen, and they "swim" up from the vagina through the cervix and uterus to meet the egg in the fallopian tube. It takes only one sperm to fertilize the egg, and that single sperm cell contains the father's genetic contribution to the baby.

Conception

When a couple has sexual intercourse the man ejaculates his semen into the woman's vagina near the cervix, the entrance to the woman's uterus. The cervix is usually blocked by cervical mucus, but this thins around the time of ovulation (when an egg is released from one of the ovaries) to allow sperm to pass through.

The sperm and egg usually meet in the fallopian tube. A single sperm penetrates and fertilizes the egg, which then travels into the uterus where it implants into the uterine lining. Pregnancy starts when the fertilized egg attaches to the uterus. Once it has implanted, hormones sustain the growing embryo, until the developing placenta can take over and nourish the pregnancy. About nine months after conception, the developing baby is ready to be born.

In the proper environment, such as the female reproductive tract beyond the cervix, sperm have a life span of up to five days. In other environments, such as the vagina, sperm live only a few hours and even less than that outside the human body, exposed to the open air. The egg, on the other hand, has a life span of only about 24 hours from the time it bursts from the ovary. Thus, fertilization can occur anytime live sperm meet up with a live egg, which can happen even if the sperm are deposited up to five days in advance of ovulation.

Take Good Care of Your Reproductive Health

- Eat a varied diet with plenty of fresh fruits and vegetables, protein-rich food such as fish (low-mercury fish), poultry, and whole grains.
- Take a multivitamin that contains folic acid.
- Avoid smoking and secondhand smoke.
- Limit alcohol and drug use.
- Exercise.
- Get adequate rest and relaxation. Avoid high stress levels.
- Keep sperm cool—sperm develop best at a temperature 2–3°C lower than the rest of the body, which is why the testes are outside the body. Wearing tight underpants or jeans can raise the temperature of the testes and lower sperm production.

Sex Determination

Chromosomes are long, stringy aggregates of genes that carry hereditary information. They are composed of DNA and proteins and are located within the nucleus of our cells. Chromosomes determine everything from hair color and eye color to gender. Whether you are a male or female depends on the presence or absence of certain chromosomes.

Human cells contain 23 pairs of chromosomes, for a total of 46. The sex chromosomes, the X and Y chromosomes, determine gender. Usually, a woman has two X chromosomes (XX) and a man has one X and one Y (XY). However, both male and female characteristics can sometimes be found in one individual, and it is possible to have XY women and XX men. If a sperm cell containing an X chromosome fertilizes an egg, the resulting zygote will be XX or female. If the sperm cell contains a Y chromosome, then the resulting zygote will be XY or male.

Sexual Orientation

Sexual orientation refers to the sex or genders to which a person is attracted and that form the focus of a person's amorous or erotic desires, fantasies, and spontaneous feelings. Sexual orientation is a natural part of human development. It remains unclear as to why individuals differ in their sexual orientation. It is known, however, that different sexual orientations have existed throughout history.

- *Heterosexual*—the focus is primarily people of the opposite sex.
- *Homosexual*—focus on people of the same sex.
- *Bisexual*—focus on potentially both or either sexes.
- *Asexual*—no sexual attraction for either sex.
- *Transsexual (TS)*—one who switches physical sexes. Primary sex change is accomplished by surgery.
- *Transvestite (TV)*—one who mainly cross dresses for pleasure in the appearance and sensation.

Although you may have had inklings of your sexual orientation in early childhood, most likely it was during adolescence that you began to determine your sexuality. Adolescence is typically a period of identity confusion in general and of sexual identity confusion in particular. It is thus not uncommon to have feelings or thoughts about being with a same-sex or different-sex partner. However, with time and experience you may come to define your sexual identity more clearly.

You may need help if:

- Your feelings about your sexuality are causing you to be depressed or anxious.
- You are unsure of what your sexual orientation is and feel that you would like to figure this out.
- You are being harassed and discriminated against.
- You and your partner are having difficulty sorting through sexual identity issues.

The Sexual Response Cycle

Sexual response is an extremely individual process. People vary in their physical, mental, and emotional reactions to sexual stimulation. However, almost all people experience certain basic physiological changes, and those changes fit with some general patterns about what happens when one is sexually aroused. Generally, there are five main stages in the sexual response cycle:

1. *Desire* (libido). This stage, in which a man or woman begins to want or "desire" sexual intimacy or gratification, may last anywhere from a moment to many years.
2. *Excitement* (arousal). This stage, which is characterized by the body's initial response to feelings of sexual desire, may last from minutes to several hours.
3. *Plateau.* The highest point of sexual excitement, plateau, generally lasts between 30 seconds and 3 minutes.
4. *Orgasm.* The peak of the plateau stage and the point at which sexual tension is released, generally lasts for less than a minute.
5. *Resolution.* The duration of this stage—the period during which the body returns to its preexcitement state—varies greatly and generally increases with age.

Sexual Dysfunction

- Erectile dysfunction
- Problems with arousal
- Hypoactive sexual desire
- Premature ejaculation
- Painful intercourse
- Sexual addiction

STDs[155]

Every year in United States, 4 million teenagers contract an STD. Abstinence is the only foolproof way of avoiding a sexually transmitted disease.

Why Young People Have High Risk of STDs

- Feeling of invulnerability
- Multiple sex partners
- Not using condoms
- Drugs and alcohol

Chlamydia is a curable infection caused by the bacteria *Chlamydia trachomatis*.

Transmission

- Chlamydia can be transmitted during vaginal, anal, and oral sex. Using latex condoms consistently and correctly—from the very beginning of sexual contact until there is no longer skin contact—reduces the risk of transmission of chlamydia.

Symptoms

- Most women and some men do *not* experience symptoms. If symptoms do occur, they usually appear within one to three weeks after infection.
- In women, if left untreated, chlamydia can cause complications such as pelvic inflammatory disease (PID) and infertility.
- In men, untreated chlamydia can cause burning and discharge during urination, inflammation of scrotal skin, and testicular swelling.

Gonorrhea is a curable infection caused by the bacteria *Neisseria gonorrhoea*.

Transmission

- Gonorrhea is transmitted during vaginal, anal, and oral sex.

Symptoms

- Many men infected with gonorrhea exhibit symptoms, whereas most women are asymptomatic. Even when women do have symptoms, they can be mistaken for a bladder infection or other vaginal infection.
- In men, symptoms usually appear within two to nine days after infection, with possible thick yellow or white pus emerging from the penis or a burning sensation.
- In women, if left untreated, gonorrhea can cause complications such as PID and infertility.
- In both genders, if left untreated, gonorrhea can lead to arthritis in joints and can attack the heart muscle, skin, and brain.

Pelvic inflammatory disease (PID) is a serious infection in the upper genital tract/reproductive organs (uterus, fallopian tubes, and ovaries) of a female. PID can be sexually transmitted or naturally occurring. It can lead to infertility in women or life-threatening complications. Women between ages 15 and 25 have the highest incidence of PID. In the United States, PID is the leading cause of infertility in women.[156]

Transmission

- Chlamydia and gonorrhea are the most common causes of PID.
- If you have an infection in the genital tract and do not get treated right away, it can cause PID.
- The infection spreads from the cervix into the uterus, fallopian tubes, and ovaries. It can take anywhere from several days to several months after being infected to develop PID.

Symptoms

- It is possible for a woman to have PID and be asymptomatic (without symptoms), or have symptoms too mild to notice, for an unknown period of time.
- Dull pain or tenderness in the lower abdomen

- Burning or pain when you urinate
- Nausea and vomiting
- Bleeding between menstrual periods
- Increased or changed vaginal discharge
- Pain during sex
- Fever and chills
- PID can also be misdiagnosed as appendicitis, ectopic pregnancy, ruptured ovarian cysts, or other problems.

Genital HPV is caused by human papillomavirus (HPV). Human papillomavirus is the name of a group of viruses that includes more than 100 different strains or types.

Some of these viruses are called "high-risk" types, and may cause abnormal Pap tests. They may also lead to cancer of the cervix, vulva, vagina, anus, or penis. Others are called "low-risk" types, and they may cause mild Pap test abnormalities or genital warts. Genital warts are single or multiple growths or bumps that appear in the genital area, and sometimes are cauliflower shaped.

Approximately 20 million people are currently infected with HPV. At least 50 percent of sexually active men and women acquire genital HPV infection at some point in their lives. By age 50, at least 80 percent of women will have acquired genital HPV infection. About 6.2 million Americans get a new genital HPV infection each year.[157]

Transmission
- The types of HPV that infect the genital area are spread primarily through genital contact.

Symptoms
- Most HPV infections have no signs or symptoms; therefore, most infected persons are unaware they are infected, yet they can transmit the virus to a sex partner.

Chancroid[158] is a curable infection caused by bacteria called *Haemophilus Ducrey*. Chancroid causes ulcers or sores, usually of the genitals. Swollen, painful lymph glands in the groin area are often associated with chancroid.

Transmission
- Left untreated, chancroid may make the transmission of HIV easier.

Chancroid is transmitted in two ways:

- sexual transmission through skin-to-skin contact with an open sore.
- nonsexual transmission when contact is made with the pus-like fluid from the ulcer.

Symptoms
- Soft painful sores or a smelly discharge. A person is considered to be infectious (able to pass the bacteria to others) when ulcers or sores are present. This means that as long as there are chancroid sores on the body, the person can spread the infection.

Crabs (also known as pubic lice)[159] are small parasites that feed on human blood. Crabs are not the same as head and body lice. Crabs are usually found on the pubic hair, but can be also be found on other parts of the body where a person has coarse hair (such as armpits, eyelashes, and facial hair). Crabs rarely infest head hair.

Transmission

- Anyone can get crabs. Having crabs does not mean a person is unclean or dirty.
- A person can get crabs during sexual contact with a person who has crabs. During the close physical contact, the crabs can move from the pubic hair of one person to the pubic hair of another. Crabs can be sexually transmitted even if there is no penetration or exchange of body fluids.
- Once off a human host, crabs can live for 24 hours, making it possible to get crabs during contact with infested bedding or clothing.

Symptoms

- The most noticeable symptom of crabs is itching. The itching usually starts about five days after a person gets crabs.

Scabies is a curable skin disease caused by the parasite *Sarcoptes scabiei*.

Transmission

- Scabies is transmitted through close physical contact with a person who is infected or prolonged contact with infested linens, furniture, or clothing.

Symptoms

- The most common symptom is itching, which usually occurs within four to six weeks after infection.
- A person is considered infectious from the time of infestation until treatment is successfully completed.

Syphilis[160] is a sexually transmitted disease caused by the bacterium *Treponema pallidum*. Pregnant women with the disease can pass it to babies. Genital sores (chancres) caused by syphilis make it easier to sexually transmit and acquire HIV infection. There is an estimated two- to five-fold increased risk of acquiring HIV infection when syphilis is present.

Transmission

- Syphilis is passed from person to person through direct contact with a syphilis sore.
- Sores occur mainly on the lips, mouth, external genitals, vagina, anus, or in the rectum.
- Transmission of the organism occurs during vaginal, anal, or oral sex.
- Syphilis cannot be spread through contact with toilet seats, doorknobs, swimming pools, hot tubs, bathtubs, shared clothing, or eating utensils.

Primary Stage

- The primary stage of syphilis is usually marked by the appearance of a single sore (called a chancre), but there may be multiple sores.
- The time between infection with syphilis and the start of the first symptom can range from 10 to 90 days (average 21 days).
- The chancre is usually firm, round, small, and painless. It appears at the spot where syphilis entered the body.
- The chancre lasts three to six weeks, and it heals without treatment. However, if adequate treatment is not administered, the infection progresses to the secondary stage.

Secondary Stage

- This stage typically starts with the development of a rash on one or more areas of the body. The rash usually does not cause itching.

- The characteristic rash of secondary syphilis may appear as rough, red, or reddish brown spots both on the palms of the hands and the bottoms of the feet.
- In addition to rashes, symptoms of secondary syphilis may include fever, swollen lymph glands, sore throat, patchy hair loss, headaches, weight loss, muscle aches, and fatigue.

Late Stage
- The latent (hidden) stage of syphilis begins when secondary symptoms disappear.
- In the late stages of syphilis, it may subsequently damage the internal organs, including the brain, nerves, eyes, heart, blood vessels, liver, bones, and joints.
- Signs and symptoms of the late stage of syphilis include difficulty coordinating muscle movements, paralysis, numbness, gradual blindness, and dementia. This damage may be serious enough to cause death.[161]

Bacterial vaginosis (BV)[162] is a condition in women in which the normal balance of bacteria in the vagina is disrupted and replaced by an overgrowth of certain bacteria. BV is the most common vaginal infection in women of childbearing age. In the United States, as many as 16 percent of pregnant women have BV.

Symptoms
- Discharge, odor, pain, itching, or burning
- Discharge, if present, is usually white or gray; it can be thin.
- Some women with BV report no signs or symptoms at all.

Some activities or behaviors can upset the normal balance of bacteria in the vagina and put women at increased risk, including:

- having a new sex partner or multiple sex partners.
- douching.
- using an intrauterine device (IUD) for contraception.

In most cases, BV causes no complications. However, some serious risks exist from BV, including:

- having BV can increase a woman's susceptibility to HIV infection if she is exposed to the HIV virus.
- having BV increases the chances that an HIV-infected woman can pass HIV to her sex partner.
- having BV has been associated with an increase in the development of pelvic inflammatory disease (PID) following surgical procedures such as a hysterectomy or an abortion.
- having BV while pregnant may put a woman at increased risk for some complications of pregnancy.
- BV can increase a woman's susceptibility to other STDs, such as chlamydia and gonorrhea.

Genital herpes is an infection of the genitals, buttocks, or anal area caused by herpes simplex virus (HSV). According to the Centers for Disease Control and Prevention, one out of five American teenagers and adults is infected with HSV type 2. Women are more commonly infected than men.[163]
There are two types of HSV:

- HSV type 1 most commonly infects the mouth and lips, causing sores known as fever blisters or cold sores. It is also an important cause of sores to the genitals.
- HSV type 2 is the usual cause of genital herpes, but it also can infect the mouth.

Transmission
- Most people get genital herpes by having sex with someone who is shedding the herpes virus either during an outbreak or during a period with no symptoms.

- Herpes can be transmitted through close contact other than sexual intercourse, through oral sex or close skin-to-skin contact, for example.
- In most people, the virus can become active and cause outbreaks several times a year. This is called a recurrence, and infected people can have symptoms.
- HSV remains in certain nerve cells of your body for life. When the virus is triggered to be active, it travels along the nerves to your skin. There, it makes more viruses and sometimes new sores near the site of the first outbreak.
- Do not have oral or genital contact in the presence of any symptoms or findings of oral herpes.

Symptoms (Outbreaks)[164]

- Symptoms might include tingling or sores near the area where the virus has entered the body, such as on the genital or rectal area, on buttocks or thighs, or occasionally on other parts of the body where the virus has entered through broken skin.
- Small red bumps appear first, develop into small blisters, and then become itchy, painful sores that might develop a crust and will heal without leaving a scar.
- Other symptoms are fever, headache, muscle aches, painful or difficult urination, vaginal discharge, and swollen glands in the groin area.
- Sometimes, the virus can become active but not cause any visible sores or any symptoms. During these times, small amounts of the virus may be shed at or near places of the first infection, in fluids from the mouth, penis, or vagina, or from barely noticeable sores. This is called asymptomatic (without symptoms) shedding. Even though you are not aware of the shedding, you can infect a sexual partner during this time. Asymptomatic shedding is an important factor in the spread of herpes.

Birth Control

Under the right circumstances, sexual relations can be a wonderful part of a relationship. Sexual relations can provide a couple with intimacy, a unique bond, and emotional fulfillment. Engaging in a sexual relationship at the wrong time, with the wrong person, or under the wrong circumstances can cause you a lot of grief. No matter what your age, some issues must be considered before becoming sexually intimate with someone. *No* method of birth control prevents pregnancy all of the time. Birth control methods can fail, but you can greatly increase a method's success rate by using it correctly all of the time. The only way to be sure you never get pregnant is to not have sex (abstinence).

The birth control method you choose should take into account:

- your overall health.
- how often you have sex.
- number of sexual partners you have.
- if you want to have children.
- how well each method works (or is effective) in preventing pregnancy.
- any potential side effects.
- your comfort level with using the method.

Following is a list of birth control methods with estimates of effectiveness, or how well they work in preventing pregnancy when used correctly, for each method:

Continuous abstinence—This means not having sexual intercourse (vaginal, anal, or oral intercourse) at any time. It is the only sure way to prevent pregnancy and protect against HIV and other STDs. This method is 100 percent effective in preventing pregnancy and STDs.

The male condom—Condoms are called barrier methods of birth control because they put up a block, or barrier, which keeps the sperm from reaching the egg. Only latex or polyurethane (because some people are allergic to latex) condoms are proven to help protect against STDs, including HIV. "Natural" or "lambskin" condoms are not recommended for STD prevention because they have tiny pores that may allow for the passage of viruses like HIV, hepatitis B, and herpes. Male condoms are 84 to 98 percent effective at preventing pregnancy.

How to Use Condoms

- Handle condoms gently.
- Store them in a cool, dry place. Long exposure to air, heat, and light makes them more breakable. Do not stash them continually in a back pocket, wallet, or glove compartment.
- Lubricate the inside and outside of the condom. (Many condoms are prelubricated.) Lubrication helps prevent rips and tears, and it increases sensitivity. Use water-based lubricants, such as K-Y jelly or AstroGlide, or silicone-based lubricants, such as Eros, with latex condoms. Oil-based lubricants like petroleum jelly, cold cream, butter, or mineral and vegetable oils damage latex.
- Put a drop or two of lubricant inside the condom.
- Pull back the foreskin, unless circumcised, before rolling on the condom.
- Place the rolled condom over the tip of the penis.
- Leave a half-inch space at the tip to collect semen.
- Pinch the air out of the tip with one hand while placing it on the penis.
- Unroll the condom over the penis with the other hand.
- Roll it all the way down to the base of the penis.
- Smooth out any air bubbles. (Friction against air bubbles can cause condom breaks.)
- Lubricate the outside of the condom.

Taking Off a Condom

- Pull out before the penis softens.
- Don't spill the semen—hold the condom against the base of the penis while you pull out.
- Throw the condom away. Condoms can only be used once.
- Wash the penis with soap and water before embracing again.

Oral contraceptives—Also called "the pill," oral contraceptives contain the hormones estrogen and progestin. They are taken daily to block the release of eggs from the ovaries. They do not protect against STDs or HIV. Oral contraceptives lighten the flow of your period and can reduce the risk of pelvic inflammatory disease (PID), ovarian cancer, benign ovarian cysts, endometrial cancer, and iron deficiency anemia. The pill is 95 to 99.9 percent effective in preventing pregnancy.

Side Effects

- Oral contraceptives increase risk of heart disease, including high blood pressure, blood clots, and blockage of the arteries, especially if you smoke.
- Some antibiotics may reduce the effectiveness of the pill. Talk to your doctor or nurse about a back-up method of birth control if she or he prescribes antibiotics.

The patch (Ortho Evra)—This is a skin patch worn on the lower abdomen, buttocks, or upper body. It releases the hormones progestin and estrogen into the bloodstream. You put on a new patch once a week for three weeks, and then do not wear a patch during the fourth week in order to have a menstrual period. The patch is 98 to 99 percent effective in preventing pregnancy, but appears to be less effective in women who weigh more than 198 pounds. It does not protect against STDs or HIV. Side effects are similar to those of the birth control pill.

Side Effects

- Breast tenderness
- Headaches
- Nausea
- Mood swings
- Weight gain (sometimes weight loss)
- Spotting and breakthrough bleeding
- Irritation at the site of application
- Blood clots
- Stroke
- Heart attacks
- Possible increased risk of cervical cancer

The hormonal vaginal contraceptive ring (NuvaRing)—The NuvaRing is a ring that releases the hormones progestin and estrogen. You squeeze the ring between your thumb and index finger and insert it into your vagina. You wear the ring for three weeks, take it out for the week that you have your period, and then put in a new ring. The ring is 98 to 99 percent effective in preventing pregnancy. Side effects are similar to those of other hormonal birth control methods.

Side Effects

- Yeast infection
- Increased vaginal discharge or irritation
- Upper respiratory tract infection
- Sinus infection
- Weight gain
- Nausea
- Spotting or breakthrough bleeding
- Headaches
- Tender breasts
- Mood swings
- Blood clots in the legs, lungs, heart, and brain
- Stroke
- Heart attack
- Gallbladder disease
- Possible increased risk of breast and ovarian cancer

IUD (intrauterine device)—An IUD is a small device that is shaped in the form of a "T." Your healthcare provider places it inside the uterus. In the United States, two types of IUDs are available: the Mirena, which continuously releases hormones for up to 5 years, and the ParaGard Copper T 380A IUD, which contains copper and can be worn for up to 12 years. Both types of IUDs primarily work in the same fashion, by preventing the fertilization of an egg. IUDs that contain hormones also work by thickening a woman's cervical mucus, thereby creating a natural barrier to sperm. The IUD has been found to be as much as 99 percent effective when inserted properly. It offers no protection against sexually transmitted diseases. The IUD is generally not recommended for women who have multiple sexual partners. The IUD may not be suitable for women who have never been pregnant before due to increased risk of expulsion. This is because of a smaller uterus and difficulty with insertion.

Side Effects

- Menstrual irregularities and spotting
- Women who use the ParaGard IUD may have anywhere from a 50 to 75 percent increase in their menstrual flow. This heavy flow may lead to anemia in some women. Additionally, women using this type of IUD may have more menstrual cramps.
- Women using the Mirena IUD are likely to experience similar side effects as those associated with the birth control pill.
- Some women have found the insertion and removal of an IUD to be painful.
- Uterine puncture
- Expulsion
- Tubal infection

The female condom (Reality)—Worn by the woman, this barrier method keeps sperm from getting into her body. It is made of polyurethane, is packaged with a lubricant, and may protect against STDs, including HIV. It can be inserted up to 24 hours prior to sexual intercourse. Female condoms are 79 to 95 percent effective at preventing pregnancy.

Side Effects

- Some people may experience irritation as a result of wearing the condom, but the risk is not as great as with latex condoms.
- Troubles inserting the condom
- In some cases, the condom may shift or slip into the vagina during sex, making the condom somewhat ineffective.
- Some people may also find that the outer ring makes sex uncomfortable, whereas others find that the outer ring is useful in stimulating the clitoris.
- Female condoms are more expensive than male condoms.

Depo-Provera—In this form of birth control, women get injections, or shots, of the hormone progestin in the buttocks or arm every three months. It does not protect against STDs or HIV. Women should not use Depo-Provera for more than two years in a row because it can cause a temporary loss of bone density that increases the longer this method is used. It is 97 percent effective in preventing pregnancy.

Side Effects

- Change in menstruation (may be lighter or heavier; shorter or longer)
- Increase in spotting and breakthrough bleeding
- Weight gain
- Dizziness
- Nervousness
- Change in libido

- Headaches
- Rash or skin discoloration
- Breast tenderness
- Depression
- Increase or decrease in facial and body hair
- Hair loss

Diaphragm, cervical cap, or shield—These are barrier methods of birth control, where the sperm are blocked from entering the cervix and reaching the egg. Before sexual intercourse, you use them with spermicide (to block or kill sperm) and place them inside your vagina to cover your cervix (the opening to your womb). You can buy spermicide gel or foam at a drug store. The diaphragm and cap are 84 to 94 percent effective in preventing pregnancy. Barrier methods must be left in place for six to eight hours after intercourse to prevent pregnancy and removed within 24 hours for the diaphragm and within 48 hours for cap and shield.

Side Effects
- People allergic to silicone or latex are likely to experience irritation and inflammation when they use these contraceptives.
- Some women may also experience frequent bladder infections.
- These methods can also increase your risk of developing toxic shock syndrome.
- It is also possible for the cervical cap or diaphragm to get pushed out of place during sex. Always check the position of your barrier device after intercourse and adjust it if you plan to have sex again.
- If you plan to use a lubricant with your latex diaphragm or cap, be sure to use one that is water-based, as oil-based lubricants can weaken latex.

Contraceptive sponge (Today Sponge)—This is a barrier method of birth control that was re-approved by the FDA in 2005. It is a soft, disc-shaped device with a loop for removal. It is made out of polyurethane foam and contains the spermicide nonoxynol-9. Before intercourse, you wet the sponge and place it, loop-side down, inside your vagina to cover the cervix. The sponge is 84 to 91 percent effective in preventing pregnancy in women who have not had a child and 68 to 80 percent effective for women who have had a child. The sponge is effective for more than one act of intercourse for up 24 hours. It needs to be left in for at least six hours after intercourse to prevent pregnancy and must be removed within 30 hours after it is inserted. The sponge does not protect against STDs or HIV.

Side Effects
- There is a risk of getting toxic shock syndrome (TSS) if the sponge is left in for more than 30 hours.
- It is possible for the sponge to shred or tear during use.
- Some women who use the sponge may experience more yeast infections.
- Women who are allergic to spermicide may experience irritation when they use a contraceptive sponge.

Surgical sterilization (tubal ligation or vasectomy)—These surgical methods are meant for people who want a permanent method of birth control. Tubal ligation or "tying tubes" is done on the woman to stop eggs from going down to her uterus where they can be fertilized. A tubal ligation is a surgical procedure whereby a woman's fallopian tubes are cut, clamped, and blocked or tied to prevent her eggs from traveling down to her uterus. It also blocks the sperm from traveling along the tube to meet the egg. The man has a vasectomy to keep sperm from going to his penis, so his ejaculate never has any sperm in it. A vasectomy involves severing the vas deferens, the tubes that carry sperm into a man's ejaculate, thereby making him infertile. The procedure takes less than 30 minutes. Surgical methods are 99.9 percent effective in preventing pregnancy.

Side Effects of Vasectomy

- Bruising and swelling (temporary)
- Infection, although this does not happen often and can usually be treated with antibiotics
- In very rare cases, the cut ends of the vas deferens grow back together

Side Effects of Tubal Ligation

- Infection and uterine perforation
- Women who have had their tubes tied and become pregnant are more likely to experience an ectopic pregnancy.
- Menstrual cycle disturbances and gynecological problems

Spermicides work by killing sperm and come in several forms—foam, gel, cream, film, suppository, or tablet. They are inserted or placed in the vagina no more than one hour before intercourse. Used alone, spermicides have a fairly high failure rate, ranging anywhere from 5 percent to as much as 59 percent. However, when used with other forms of birth control, spermicides may help increase their efficacy. All spermicides have sperm-killing chemicals in them. Some spermicides also have an ingredient called *nonoxynol-9* that may increase the risk of HIV infection when used because it irritates the tissue in the vagina and anus, which can cause the virus to enter the body more freely.

Emergency contraceptives are methods of *preventing* pregnancy *after* unprotected sexual intercourse. Emergency contraception is often called "the morning after pill," but this is misleading because emergency contraception can be used *before* the morning after or up to five days after. Emergency contraceptives *do not* protect against sexually transmitted infections. Emergency contraception can be used when a condom breaks, after a sexual assault, or any time unprotected sexual intercourse occurs.

Emergency contraceptives include:

1. Emergency contraceptive pills (ECPs) are sometimes wrongly called the "morning after pill." This is wrong because ECPs are never taken as one pill, the "morning after." They are taken in two doses, 12 hours apart. They work best if taken within 72 hours of unprotected vaginal intercourse. ECPs contain higher doses of hormones than those contained in birth control pills.

   - **Ella:** The Food and Drug Administration approved a controversial new form of emergency contraception that can prevent a pregnancy as many as five days after sex. Critics argue that it was misleading to approve ella as a contraceptive because the drug could also be used to induce an abortion. Ella can cut the chances of becoming pregnant by about two-thirds for at least 120 hours after a contraceptive failure or unprotected sex, studies have shown.

2. The copper-T intrauterine device (the Copper-T IUD), which is shaped like a "T" and placed inside the uterus (or womb) by a health-care provider. This must be done within seven days after unprotected vaginal intercourse.

Emergency contraception keeps a woman from getting pregnant by stopping:

- ovulation, or stopping the ovaries from releasing eggs that can be fertilized.
- fertilization, or stopping the egg from being fertilized by the sperm.
- implantation, or stopping a fertilized egg from attaching itself to the wall of the uterus.

Abortion Pills

"Abortion pills" (Mifeprex [*mifepristone*], also called RU-486) work after a woman becomes pregnant—after a fertilized egg attaches to the wall of the uterus. These pills cause the uterus to expel the egg, ending the pregnancy. The first dose of mifepristone works by blocking the body's production of progesterone, which is needed to help keep the uterine lining suitable for the embryo. Without the progesterone, the uterine lining thins and the pregnancy is ended. The second dose will cause uterine contractions, thereby forcing the body to expel the contents of the uterus. Abortion pills are effective 96 to 97 percent of the time. They can cause hemorrhaging.

Surgical Abortion

Three types of surgical abortion are performed: manual vacuum aspiration, dilation and suction curettage, and dilation and evacuation.

Manual vacuum aspiration: This type of abortion can be done up to 10 weeks after a woman's last menstrual period. In this procedure, a syringe is used to suction out the embryo. The actual procedure takes about 10 minutes plus prep and recovery time. Local anesthetic is usually given.

Dilation and suction curettage (D&C): This type of abortion is performed between 6 and 14 weeks after a woman's last menstrual period. This type of abortion involves a mechanical suction device to remove the contents of the uterus, including the embryo or fetus. A curette is then used to scrape the walls of the uterus in order to make sure everything has been cleaned out. Local or general anesthetic may be administered and the procedure takes about 10 minutes plus prep and recovery time.

Dilation and evacuation: Performed from the 13th week of pregnancy on, this type of abortion involves slowly opening the cervix to allow room for forceps, a suction device, and curette. The procedure is very similar to a D&C but forceps are also used to remove the fetus. When an abortion is done late in pregnancy, it is usually for medical reasons.

Risks of Surgical Abortions

It's very important that a woman goes to a licensed clinic to lessen the risks of surgical abortions.

- Incomplete abortion
- Infection
- Extremely heavy bleeding
- Allergic reaction to medication
- Uterine blood clots
- Torn or severed cervix
- Uterine puncture damaging other organs
- Death
- Emotional disturbances

Access to Abortion

In the United States, abortion laws vary from state to state. Depending on your age and which state you live in, there may be laws in place that prevent you from having an abortion or require you to get parental permission if you are under a certain age. There may also be mandatory education or waiting periods before an abortion can be done. Additionally, some clinics may require that you pay them up front while others offer a payment plan. In some instances, Medicaid covers the cost of an abortion. Women living in Canada who have an abortion in a hospital will have the cost covered by provincial health care.[165]

Teen Pregnancy

About 35 percent of girls in the United States get pregnant at least once by age 20. Many teens say they are concerned about pregnancy, but still think "it can't happen to me." But it does—to 900,000 girls every year. Research suggests that early sexual experience among adolescents has been associated with depression, suicide, alcohol, and drug use.[166] And the number-one reason teen guys and girls give for not using protection is that they weren't planning to have sex and that it "just happened."[167] The United States still leads the fully industrialized world in teen pregnancy and birth rates, by a wide margin. In fact, the U.S. rates are nearly double Great Britain's, at least 4 times those of France and Germany, and more than 10 times that of Japan.[168]

Consequences of Teen Motherhood

- Less likely to complete high school
- Dependence on welfare
- Single parenthood
- More likely to have more children sooner on a limited income
- More likely to abuse or neglect the child

Risks to Children of Teen Mothers

- Growing up without a father
- Low birth weight and prematurity
- School failure
- Mental retardation
- Insufficient health care
- Abuse and neglect
- Poverty and welfare dependence

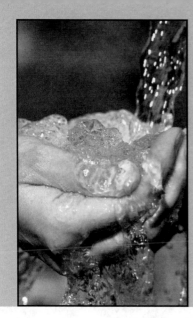

Chapter 11
Infectious Diseases

Infectious Diseases

Infectious diseases are caused by microscopic organisms—including bacteria, viruses, fungi and animal parasites—that penetrate the body's natural barriers and multiply to create symptoms that can range from mild to deadly.

A *pathogen* or *infectious agent* is a biological agent that causes disease or illness to its host. The human body has many natural defenses against some of the more common pathogens in the form of the human immune system and by some "helpful" bacteria present in the human body's normal flora. However, if the immune system or "good" bacteria is damaged in any way (such as by chemotherapy, human immunodeficiency virus [HIV], or antibiotics being taken to kill other pathogens), pathogenic bacteria that was being held at bay can proliferate and cause harm to the host.

Bacteria are a major group of living organisms. Most are microscopic and unicellular.

A *virus* is a submicroscopic parasite that infects cells in biological organisms. Viruses are not cells. They consist of one or more molecules of DNA or RNA, which contain the virus's genes surrounded by a protein coat. They can reproduce only by invading and controlling other cells because they lack the cellular machinery for self-reproduction.

A *parasite* is an organism that spends a significant portion of its life in or on the living tissue of a host organism and that causes harm to the host without immediately killing it.

Modes of Infection

Common ways in which infectious agents enter the body are through:

- Skin contact
- Inhalation of airborne microbes
- Ingestion of contaminated food or water
- Bites from vectors such as ticks or mosquitoes that carry and transmit organisms
- Sexual contact and transmission from mothers to their unborn children via the birth canal and placenta

Prevention

Immunization[169]

- Modern vaccines are among our most effective strategies to prevent disease. Many devastating diseases can now be prevented through appropriate immunization programs.
- In the United States, it is recommended that all children be vaccinated against diphtheria, pertussis (whooping cough), tetanus, polio, measles, rubella (German measles), mumps, Haemophilus influenza type B (a common cause of pneumonia and meningitis in infants), hepatitis B, varicella (chickenpox) and influenza.
- Travelers to foreign countries may require vaccinations against yellow fever, cholera, typhoid fever, or hepatitis A and B.

Public Health Measures

- Measures that assure clean water supplies, adequate sewage treatment, and sanitary handling of food and milk also are important to control the spread of infectious disease.

Personal Prevention Measures

- Hand washing
- Immunization
- Pasteurization
- Sex protection

Treatment

The development of antibiotics and other antimicrobials has played an important role in the fight against infectious diseases, but some microorganisms develop resistance to the drugs used against them.

How Your Immune System Works

- Because of poor diets, stress, and inactivity many children and adults have immune systems that don't operate at peak efficiency.
- White blood cells are the body's infantry, the hard-working soldiers on the front lines. These cells patrol the body's bloodstream, preventing germs from entering cells.
- When germs try to hide from the white cells, specialized units of white cells, called *macrophages* ("big eaters"), search the body to gobble up harmful invaders.
- Suppose a flu virus enters your body, multiplies rapidly, and threatens to overwhelm the circulating white cell army; the immune system deploys specialized cells that will fight the invaders. These include T-lymphocytes (white cells that originate in the thymus, a tiny gland in front of the heart) and killer lymphocytes.
- If a germ enters the body through a break in the skin or an infection in the throat, the white cells send out chemical messengers that quickly mobilize reinforcements and direct them to the area of infection.
- Once they reach the battle, these cells produce chemical fighters, known as cytokines (meaning molecules that move to the cells).
- Cytokines dilate the blood vessels, causing more blood flow and enabling more white cell police to enter the infected area of battle.

218

- Another task of these cytokine messengers is to tell the body to conserve supplies, such as important nutrients that are needed to win the infection battle.
- The army of white cells and chemical messengers has a number of chemical weapons available. They can shoot gamma-interferon into the enemy. This substance interferes with the body's ability to reproduce itself.
- Another special group of white cells, called B-cells, produces chemicals called antibodies, which seek out and attach themselves to specific germs.
- Some of these antibodies, called immunoglobulins, poke holes in the germs, so that in essence they "bleed" to death.
- Others act like chemical glue, making the germs stick together so that they can be rounded up easily by the white blood cells.

How Immunizations Work

- If the same or a similar germ tries to attack again, the immune system is ready for it. It recognizes the invader and destroys it.
- The small dose of killed virus given in an immunization sets up a training exercise for the immune army.

Two Broad Categories of Immune System Disorders

1. *Immunodeficiency* (lacking or deficient)—when the immune system does not recognize invaders as being undesirable and therefore does not mobilize to destroy them.
   - Pneumonia, thrush, diarrhea, AIDS/HIV, infections, cancer, severe acute respiratory syndrome
2. *Autoimmunity* (excessive or self-destruction)—when the immune system fails to recognize "self" as friendly and mounts an attack on itself.
   - Hashimoto's thyroiditis, pernicious anemia, diabetes I, rheumatoid arthritis, lupus, multiple sclerosis, graves disease, psoriasis, eczema, cushing's, fibromyalgia, scleroderma

How to Boost Your Immunity

Protecting the immune system is a vital part of living longer, feeling younger, and being healthy.

1. *Handwashing.* Washing your hands with soap and water as soon as you come home, and always before you eat, greatly reduces your exposure to bacterial and viral infections. In case you cannot wash with soap and water when you are away from home, carry some alcohol-based hand wipes with you to control microbial exposure and transmission.
2. *Physical activity.* Regular exercise and physical activity strengthens your immune system, cardiovascular system, heart, muscles, and bones. It also stimulates the release of endorphins; improves mental functioning, concentration/attention and cognitive performance; and lowers cholesterol, blood pressure, cortisol, and other stress hormones. Three 10-minute workout sessions during the day are just as effective as one 30-minute workout, and a lot easier to fit into a busy schedule.
3. *Yoga and stretching.* The slow movements and controlled postures of yoga improve muscle strength, flexibility, range of motion, balance, breathing, and blood circulation and promotes mental focus, clarity, and calmness. Stretching also reduces mental and physical stress, tension, and anxiety; promotes good sleep; lowers blood pressure; and slows down your heart rate.
4. *High-Nutrient Diet.*
   - *Avoid too much fat*—Obesity can lead to a depressed immune system. It can affect the ability of white blood cells to multiply, produce antibodies, and rush to the site of an infection.

- *Avoid overdosing on sugar*—Eating or drinking 40 grams (8 tbsp.) of sugar, the equivalent of one 12-ounce can of soda, can reduce the ability of white blood cells to kill germs by 40 percent. The immune-suppressing effect of sugar starts less than 30 minutes after ingestion and may last for 5 hours. In contrast, the ingestion of complex carbohydrates and fiber has a positive effect on the immune system.
- *Eat foods rich in antioxidants* (like vitamins A, C, E and lycopene), *Omega-3 fatty acids, and folate.*
  - *Antioxidants* fight and neutralize free radicals, which are molecules that damage cells and cause heart disease, cancer, and premature aging.
    - Food sources: pumpkin, sweet potatoes, carrots, kale, grapefruit (red and pink), blueberries, strawberries, watermelon, cantaloupe, oranges, peppers (red and green), tomatoes, broccoli, sunflower seeds, almonds, and olive oil.
  - *Omega-3 fatty acids* (a polyunsaturated fat) have anti-inflammatory, cardiovascular-enhancing and immune-regulating properties. They are helpful in preventing and controlling high cholesterol, hypertension, heart disease, stroke, cancer, diabetes, depression, and inflammatory and autoimmune disorders.
    - Food sources: ground flax seeds, walnuts, soybeans, and pumpkin seeds.
  - *Folate* prevents age-related cognitive decline and damage to blood vessels and brain cells by lowering homocysteine levels. It also ensures DNA integrity (important as we age and when pregnant) and promotes healthy red blood cells.
    - Food sources: dark green leafy vegetables (turnip greens, mustard greens, spinach, romaine lettuce, collard greens), beans, legumes, asparagus, brussels sprouts, beets, and okra.

5. *Sleep.* A chronic lack of sleep can leave you feeling sluggish, irritable, forgetful, accident-prone, and cause difficulty concentrating or coping with life's daily aggravations. Long-term sleep loss can also result in heart disease, stroke, hypertension, depression, and anxiety. Sleep time is when your body and immune system do most of their repairs and rejuvenation. Strive to get seven to eight hours of sleep each night.

6. *Stop smoking.* Tobacco smoke impairs the immune system. The smokers are more prone to infections. It takes longer to get over an illness. Smoking harms nearly every organ in the body. Many of the 4,000 chemicals in tobacco smoke are chemically active and trigger profound and potentially fatal changes in the body.

7. *Avoid excess alcohol.* Excessive alcohol intake can harm the body's immune system in two ways. First, it produces an overall nutritional deficiency, depriving the body of valuable immune-boosting nutrients. Second, alcohol, like sugar, consumed in excess can reduce the ability of white cells to kill germs. One drink does not appear to bother the immune system, but three or more drinks do.

8. *Positive thinking/visualization and meditation.* Optimism can counteract the negative impact stress, tension, and anxiety have on your immune system and well-being. Having a positive attitude, finding the good in what life throws your way, and looking at the bright side of things enhances your ability to effectively manage stress. Visualization and meditation are effective ways of counteracting stress and calming down your nervous system.

9. *Laughter and humor. Laughter is the best medicine.* Laughing reduces stress hormones such as adrenaline (epinephrine) and cortisol. It also benefits your immune system by increasing the number and activity of "natural killer" T-cells. These cells act as the first line of defense against viral attacks and damaged cells.

10. *Music.* Listening to your favorite music is a great method of reducing stress and relieving anxiety. Pay attention to how you feel when you hear a particular song or genre of music, and keep listening to the ones that produce a relaxing effect.

Common Cold[170]

- The cold is the most commonly occurring illness in the entire world, with more than 1 billion colds per year reported in the United States alone. The common cold is a self-limiting illness caused by any one of more than 200 viruses.
- The primary means of spreading a cold is through hand-to-hand contact or from objects that have been touched by someone with a cold.

Symptoms

- The common cold produces mild symptoms usually lasting only 5–10 days.
- Runny nose
- Sneezing
- Nasal and sinus blockage
- Headache
- Sore throat
- Cough

Treatment

- To date, no specific cure has been found for the group of viruses that cause the common cold.
- Antibiotics kill bacteria, not viruses, and are of no use in treating a cold.
- Congestion: Drink plenty of fluids to help break up your congestion. Drinking water or juice will prevent dehydration and keep your throat moist. Inhaled steam may ease your congestion and drippy nose.
- A warm saltwater gargle can relieve a scratchy throat.

Influenza

Commonly called "the flu," influenza is a highly contagious viral infection of the respiratory tract.

- Influenza is spread from person to person through airborne droplets from the nose or throat of an infected person.
- Compared with most other viral respiratory infections, such as the common cold, influenza infection often causes a more severe illness.
- Most people who get influenza recover completely in one to two weeks, but some people develop serious complications, such as pneumonia.
- The elderly and persons with chronic health problems are most at risk for developing serious complications after influenza infection.

Symptoms

Symptoms typically appear one to five days after infection.

- Abrupt fever
- Muscle aches
- Severe tiredness
- Cough
- Sore throat

- Runny or stuffy nose
- Headache

Tuberculosis (TB)[171]

TB is a serious, reemerging bacterial illness that usually affects the lungs.

- TB bacteria are spread from person to person through the air.
- There are two forms of TB: (1) TB infection, and (2) TB disease (active TB). Most people with TB have infection. People with TB infection have no symptoms and cannot spread TB to others. People with TB disease have symptoms and can spread TB to others.
- People with TB disease of the lung spray the bacteria into the air when they cough, sneeze, talk, or laugh. People nearby can breathe in the bacteria and become infected.
- When a person breathes in TB bacteria, they lodge in the lungs and begin to multiply. From there, the bacteria sometimes move through the blood to other parts of the body, such as the kidneys, joints, and brain. In most cases, the infection is kept in check by the body's immune system. In about 10 percent of cases, however, the infection breaks out into active TB disease at some point during the life of the infected person.
- TB infection is diagnosed by a skin test. A small needle is used to put some fluid, called tuberculin, under the skin on the inside of the arm. After two to three days, the amount of skin swelling around the test area is measured. A positive reaction usually means that the person has TB infection. TB disease is diagnosed by a chest x-ray or a test of a sputum sample.
- People with TB infection can take medicine to keep them from getting TB disease.
- People with TB disease can usually be cured with anti-TB drugs. To be effective, the drugs must be taken exactly as prescribed. Some new strains of TB are resistant to many anti-TB drugs.

Symptoms

Symptoms of TB disease depend on where in the body the TB bacteria are multiplying. TB bacteria usually multiply in the lungs. TB in the lungs can cause:

- A bad cough that lasts longer than two weeks
- Chest pain
- Coughing up blood or sputum (phlegm from deep inside the lungs)
- Other symptoms are: weakness or tiredness, weight loss, chills, fever, and night sweats

Preventing TB involves: (1) keeping people from becoming infected with TB, (2) keeping people with TB infection from getting TB disease, (3) treating people with TB disease, and (4) implementing precautions in institutional settings to reduce the risk of TB transmission.

Chronic Fatigue Syndrome (CFS)

CFS is a debilitating disorder characterized by profound tiredness.

- The cause of chronic fatigue syndrome has not yet been identified.
- People with chronic fatigue syndrome suffer from exhaustion and are forced to function at a much lower level of activity than they did when healthy. Some people eventually recover, but others get progressively worse.
- There is no known treatment or cure for chronic fatigue syndrome.
- The recovery time varies widely. Some people eventually make a full recovery, but others seem to get progressively worse. People with chronic fatigue syndrome often have alternating times of illness and relatively good health. Some improve a bit but never fully recover.

Symptoms

- Profound tiredness—people with chronic fatigue syndrome often become exhausted from only light physical activity and must function at a much lower level of activity than they did when healthy.
- Other symptoms are weakness, muscle aches and pains, excessive sleep, fever, sore throat, tender lymph glands, forgetfulness, confusion, difficulty concentrating, and depression.

Group A Streptococcus

This bacterium is commonly found in the throat and on the skin.

- Group A strep bacteria can cause a range of infections, from relatively mild sore throats and skin infections to life-threatening invasive disease.
- Group A strep bacteria are spread by direct person-to-person contact.
- The bacteria are carried in discharges from the nose or throat of an infected person and in infected wounds or sores on the skin.
- The bacteria are usually spread when infected secretions come in contact with the mouth, nose, or eyes of an uninfected person. They can also enter the body through a cut or scrape.
- Group A strep infections can usually be treated with antibiotics.

Symptoms

- Painful throat
- Swollen glands
- Sometimes a fever is present
- Bright red tonsils and throat
- White or yellow spots at back of throat
- A swollen, tender neck
- Weakness
- Loss of appetite

Prevention of group A strep infections: (1) wash hands thoroughly and often, (2) get a throat culture for a sore throat with fever, and (3) keep wounds clean and seek medical care for infected wounds with fever.

Pneumococcal Disease[172]

Pneumococcal disease refers to infections caused by the bacterium *Streptococcus pneumoniae*, also called the pneumococcus.

- Pneumococcal disease is the leading cause of death from vaccine-preventable bacterial disease in the United States.
- Serious illnesses caused by the pneumococcus include *pneumonia* (infection of the lungs), bloodstream infection, and *meningitis* (infection of the lining of the brain and spinal cord).
- Pneumococcal meningitis can result in permanent damage to the brain and nervous system, learning deficits, and deafness.
- The bacteria spreads from person to person through secretions from the nose, mouth, and throat.

Symptoms of Pneumonia

- Fever
- Difficulty breathing
- Cough
- Chest pain

Symptoms of Bacterial Meningitis

- Fever
- Sleepiness or irritability
- Headache
- Vomiting
- Seizures
- Loss of consciousness

Viral Meningitis

Viral meningitis is a relatively common but rarely serious infection of the fluid in the spinal cord and the fluid that surrounds the brain.

- Viral meningitis is caused by any of a number of different viruses, many of which are associated with other diseases.
- Mosquito-borne viruses can also cause viral meningitis.
- There is no specific treatment for viral meningitis. The illness is usually mild and clears up in about a week.
- Prevention centers on washing hands thoroughly and often and avoiding mosquito bites.
- Symptoms include fever, headache, stiff neck, and tiredness. Rash, sore throat, and vomiting can also occur.
- Symptoms generally appear within one week of exposure. Illness usually lasts less than 10 days, and people usually recover completely without complications.

Mononucleosis

Sometimes called "mono" or "the kissing disease," mononucleosis is an infection that is usually caused by the Epstein-Barr virus (EBV).

- EBV is very common, and most people have been exposed to the virus at some time in childhood. Not everyone who is exposed to the virus develops the symptoms of mono.
- Although EBV is the most common cause of mono, other viruses, such as *cytomegalovirus*, can cause a similar illness. Like EBV, cytomegalovirus stays in the body for life and may not cause any symptoms.
- One common way to "catch" mono is by kissing someone who has been infected.
- You can also get mononucleosis through other types of direct contact with saliva from someone infected with the virus, such as by sharing a cigarette, a drink, or an eating utensil.
- Some people who have the virus in their bodies never have any symptoms, but it is still possible to pick up the virus from them.
- There is no cure for mononucleosis, but the illness will go away by itself, usually in three to four weeks.

Symptoms usually begin to appear four to seven weeks after infection with the virus and include:

- Constant fatigue
- Fever
- Sore throat
- Loss of appetite
- Swollen lymph nodes
- Headaches
- Sore muscles
- Skin rash
- Abdominal pain

Lyme Disease

Lyme disease is caused by a bacterium called *Borrelia burgdorferi,* which is transmitted by the bites of infected ticks.

- A tick can be removed by grasping its head with thin-tipped tweezers and pulling straight out without jerking or twisting.

Symptoms

- An expanding red rash, which starts at the site of the tick bite, may appear a few days to a few weeks after the tick bite.
- Fever, headache, muscle aches, and joint pain may also occur. If it goes untreated, later symptoms can include recurring rash, joint pain, heart disease, and nervous system disorders.
- Treatment with oral antibiotics during the early stages of Lyme disease reduces the likelihood of later symptoms.

Prevention

- When working or hiking in areas with ticks, wear light-colored long-sleeved shirts, long pants tucked into socks, and closed shoes (not sandals).
- Use tick repellent spray on clothing.
- After outdoor activities, wash clothing and check each person's body, including hair, for ticks.
- Pets can also get Lyme disease, so check them too.

Hepatitis A

Hepatitis A is a liver disease caused by the hepatitis A virus (HAV).

- In the United States, hepatitis A can occur in situations ranging from isolated cases of disease to widespread epidemics.
- Good personal hygiene and proper sanitation can help prevent hepatitis A.
- Vaccines are also available for long-term prevention of hepatitis A virus infection in persons 12 months of age and older.
- HAV is found in the stool (feces) of persons with hepatitis A.
- HAV is usually spread from person to person by putting something in the mouth (even though it may look clean) that has been contaminated with the stool of a person with hepatitis A.

Symptoms
- Jaundice
- Fatigue
- Abdominal pain
- Loss of appetite
- Nausea, vomiting
- Joint pain

Hepatitis B (HBV)

HBV is a serious disease caused by a virus that attacks the liver.
- The virus can cause lifelong infection, cirrhosis (scarring) of the liver, liver cancer, liver failure, and death. Occurs when blood from an infected person enters the body of a person who is not infected.
- HBV is spread through having sex with an infected person without using a condom (the efficacy of latex condoms in preventing infection with HBV is unknown, but their proper use may reduce transmission); by sharing drugs, needles, or "works" when "shooting" drugs; through needlesticks or sharps exposures on the job; or from an infected mother to her baby during birth.

Symptoms
- Jaundice
- Fatigue
- Abdominal pain
- Loss of appetite
- Nausea, vomiting
- Joint pain

Hepatitis C (HCV)

HCV occurs when blood from an infected person enters the body of a person who is not infected.
- HCV is spread through sharing needles or "works" when "shooting" drugs, through needlesticks or sharps exposures on the job, or from an infected mother to her baby during birth.

Symptoms
- Jaundice
- Fatigue
- Dark urine
- Abdominal pain
- Loss of appetite
- Nausea

Long-Term Effects
- Chronic infection: 55 to 85 percent of infected persons
- Chronic liver disease: 70 percent of chronically infected persons

- Deaths from chronic liver disease: 1 to 5 percent of infected persons may die
- Leading indication for liver transplant

Prevention

There is no vaccine to prevent hepatitis C.

- Do not shoot drugs.
- Do not share personal care items that might have blood on them (razors, toothbrushes).
- If you are a healthcare or public safety worker, always follow routine barrier precautions and safely handle needles and other sharps.
- Consider the risks if you are thinking about getting a tattoo or body piercing.
- If you are having sex with more than one steady sex partner, use latex condoms correctly and every time to prevent the spread of sexually transmitted diseases.
- If you are HCV positive, do not donate blood, organs, or tissue.

HIV/AIDS[173]

Human immunodeficiency virus (HIV) is the virus that causes AIDS, or acquired immunodeficiency syndrome. HIV harms the body's immune system by attacking certain cells, known as helper T-cells or CD4 cells, which defend the body against illness. CDC's definition of AIDS includes all HIV-infected people who have fewer than 200 CD4+ T-cells per cubic millimeter of blood. (Healthy adults usually have CD4+ T-cell counts of 1,000 or more.)

At the end of 2003, an estimated 1,039,000 to 1,185,000 persons in the United States were living with HIV/AIDS, with 24 to 27 percent undiagnosed and unaware of their HIV infection.[174] Approximately 40 million people worldwide are living with HIV.

The epidemic is growing most rapidly among minority populations and is a leading killer of African American males ages 25 to 44. According to the CDC, AIDS affects nearly seven times more African Americans and three times more Hispanics than whites. The rate of AIDS among black women is 27 times the rate among white women.[175]

People diagnosed with AIDS may get life-threatening diseases called *opportunistic infections*, which are caused by microbes such as viruses or bacteria that usually do not make healthy people sick. In people with AIDS, these infections are often severe and sometimes fatal because the immune system is so ravaged by HIV that the body cannot fight off certain bacteria, viruses, fungi, parasites, and other microbes.

AIDS stands for **a**cquired **i**mmuno**d**eficiency **s**yndrome.[176]

Acquired means that the disease is not hereditary but develops after birth from contact with a disease-causing agent (in this case, HIV).

Immunodeficiency means that the disease is characterized by a weakening of the immune system.

Syndrome refers to a group of symptoms that collectively indicate or characterize a disease. In the case of AIDS this can include the development of certain infections and/or cancers, as well as a decrease in the number of certain cells in a person's immune system.

Transmission

- HIV is spread most commonly by having unprotected sex with an infected partner. The virus can enter the body through the lining of the vagina, penis, rectum, or mouth during sex.
- Sharing drug needles or syringes
- HIV-infected women to their babies before or during birth, or through breastfeeding after birth

Symptoms

Many people will not have any symptoms when they first become infected with HIV. Some have a flu-like illness within a month or two after exposure to the virus.

- Fever
- Headache
- Tiredness
- Enlarged lymph nodes (glands of the immune system easily felt in the neck and groin)

Prevention

- Speak openly with partners about safer sex techniques and HIV status.
- If you don't know your status, get an HIV test to protect yourself and others.
- Use a latex condom with each oral, anal, or vaginal sexual encounter. *Those with latex allergies should use latex-free condoms.*
- Do not share needles or syringes.
- HIV-infected pregnant women should get into regular prenatal and postpartum care.
- HIV-infected women should not breastfeed.

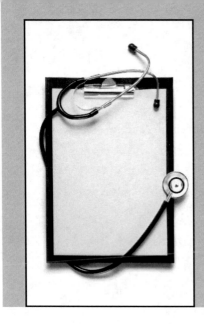

Notes

1. World Health Organization. "Constitution of the World Health Organization." *Chronicle of the World Health Organization*. Geneva, Switzerland: WHO, 1947.

2. U.S. Department of Health and Human Services. *Mental Health: A Report of the Surgeon General: Executive Summary*. Rockville, MD: U.S. Department of Health and Human Services, Substance Abuse and Mental Health Service Administration, Center for Mental Health Services, National Institute of Health, National Institute of Mental Health, 1999.

3. National Center for Statistics and Analysis. "Top 10 Leading Causes of Death in the US for 2002." http://www.nhtsa.dot.gov.

4. Ibid.

5. Healthy People 2010 Fact Sheet. "Healthy People in Healthy Communities." http://www.health.gov.healthypeople.

6. Scanlan, James. "Race and Mortality." *Society*, Vol. 37, No. 2, January 2000.

7. Guyer, Bernard, et al. "Annual Summary of Vital Statistics: Trends in the Health of Americans During the 20th Century." *Pediatrics*, Vol. 106, No. 6, December 2000.

8. Milansky, Aubrey. *Your Genetic Destiny*. New York: Perseus Publishing, 2001.

9. Vitucci, Jeff. "The State of Hispanic Health." *Hispanic Business*, Vol. 21, No. 6, June 1999.

10. World Health Organization. 2004. Why Gender and Health? http://www.who.int/gender/genderandhealth/en.

11. Hales, Dianne. *An Invitation to Health*, 11th ed. Belmont, CA: Thomson/Wadsworth, 2005.

12. National Mental Heath Association. "Mental Health Fact Sheets." http://www.nmha.org/.

13. Ibid.

14. Ibid.

15. Ibid.

16. Ibid.

17. National Mental Health Association. "Depression Fact Sheet." http://www.nmha.org/infoctr/factsheets/21.cfm.

18. National Institute of Mental Health. "The Numbers Count: Mental Illness in America." *Science on Our Minds Fact Sheet Series*. http://www.nimh.nih.gov/publicat/numbers.cfm.

19. Hales, *An Invitation to Health*, p. 57.

20. Ibid.

21. Ibid.

22. Weitzstein, Cheryl. "Preventing Suicide." *Insight in the News*, Vol. 16, No. 16, May 1, 2000.

23. Ibid.

24. Hales, *An Invitation to Health*, p. 62.

25. National Mental Health Association. "Suicide Fact Sheet." http://www.nmha.org/infoctr/factsheets/51.cfm.

26. Ho, Beng-Choon, et al. "Schizophrenia and Other Psychotic Disorders." In *Textbook of Clinical Psychiatry*, 4th ed. Washington, DC: American Psychiatric Publishing, Inc., 2003, p. 379.

27. National Mental Health Association. "Seasonal Affective Disorder Fact Sheet." http://www.nmha.org/infoctr/factsheets/27.cfm.

28. National Institute of Mental Health. "What Is Social Phobia?" http://www.nimh.nih.gov/healthinformation/socialphobiamenu.cfm.

29. Insel, P., and Roth, W., eds. 2006. *Core Concepts in Health*, 10th ed. New York: McGraw-Hill.

30. Dunn, A.L., M.H. Trivedi, J.B. Kampert, C.G. Clark, and H.O. Chambliss. "Exercise Treatment for Depression—Efficacy and Dose Response." *American Journal of Preventive Medicine*. January, 2005.

31. http://www.google.com/search?hl=en&lr=&client=firefox-a&rls=org.mozilla:en-US:official&oi=defmore&defl=en&q=defin:Hormone.

32. http://www.alz.org/Resources/Glossary.asp.

33. Newman, E. *No More Test Anxiety*. Los Angeles, CA: Learning Skills Publications, 1996.

34. http://www.contemplativemind.org/practices/subnav/mindfulness.htm.

35. Ibid.

36. Jacobson, E. *Progressive relaxation*. Chicago: University of Chicago Press, 1938.

37. http://www.ship.edu/~cgboeree/musclerelaxation.html.

38. Booth, Frank, et al. "Physiologists Claim SEDS Is Second Greatest Threat to US Public Health." *Medical Letter on the CDC & FDA*, June 24, 2001.

39. "Physical Activity and Health: Adults," a Report of the Surgeon General, President's Council on Physical Fitness and Sports, http://www.cdc.gov.

40. Grubbs, L., and J. Carter. "The Relationship of Perceived Benefit and Barriers to Reported Exercise Behaviors in College Undergraduates." *Family and Community Health*, Vol. 25, No. 2, July 2002, p. 76.

41. Prochaska, J.O., and C.C. DiClemente. "Transtheoretical Therapy Toward a More Integrative Model of Change." *Psychotherapy: Theory, Research and Practice*, Vol. 19, No. 3, pp. 276–287.

42. Prochaska, J.O., J.C. Norcross, and C.C. DiClemente. *Changing for Good*. New York: William Morrow, 1994.

43. American Heart Association. "A Statement on Exercise: Benefits and Recommendations for Physical Activity Programs for All Americans." *Circulation*, Vol. 91, p. 580.

44. American College of Sports Medicine. *ACSM's Guidelines for Exercise Testing and Prescription.* Baltimore, MD: Lippincott Williams and Wilkins, 2000.

45. American College of Sports Medicine. "Position Stand: The Recommended Quality and Quantity of Exercise for Developing and Maintaining Cardiorespiratory and Muscular Fitness, and Flexibility in Healthy Adults." *Medicine and Science in Sports and Exercise*, Vol. 30, 1998, pp. 975–991.

46. American College of Sports Medicine. http://www.acsm.org.

47. Borg, G. A. "Psychophysical Basis of Perceived Exertion." *Medicine and Science in Sports and Exercise*, Vol. 14, No. 5, 2003, pp. 377–381.

48. Ibid.

49. American College of Sports Medicine. "The Recommended Quantity and Quality of Exercise for Developing and Maintaining Cardiorespiratory and Muscular Fitness and Flexibility in Healthy Adults." *Medicine and Science in Sports and Exercise*, Vol. 30, No. 6, 1998, pp. 975–991.

50. Shrier, I., and K. Gossal. "Myths and Truths of Stretching." *Physician and Sports Medicine*, Vol. 28, No. 8, 2000, pp. 57–63.

51. Thygerson, A. *Fit to Be Well: Essential Concepts.* Sudbury, MA: Jones and Bartlett, 2005, p. 52.

52. Ibid.

53. Pfeiffer, R., and B. Mangus. *Concepts of Athletic Training*, 4th ed. Sudbury, MA: Jones and Bartlett, 2004, p. 265.

54. American Heart Association. http://www.americanheart.org/presenter.jhtml?identifier=2155.

55. American Council on Fitness. http://www.acefitness.org/fitfacts/fitfacts_display.aspx?itemid=57.

56. American Heart Association. http://www.americanheart.org.

57. *USA Today*, January 8, 2006. http://www.usatoday.com/news/health/2006-01-08-heart-nine-factors_x.htm.

58. American Heart Association. "Women and Heart Disease." http://www.americanheart.org/presenter.jhtml?identifier=2876.

59. American Heart Association. http://www.americanheart.org/presenter.jhtml?identifier=3053#Heart_Attack.

60. *New York Times*, January 9, 2006. http://www.nytimes.com/2006/01/09/nyregion/nyregionspecial5/09diabetes.html?ei=5094&en=3a1180cac87d23c8&hp=&ex=1136869200&oref=login&partner=homepage&pagewanted=print.

61. *New York Times*, January 9, 2006. http://www.nytimes.com/2006/01/09/nyregion/nyregionspecial5/09diabetes.html?ei=5094&en=3a1180cac87d23c8&hp=&ex=1136869200&oref=login&partner=homepage&pagewanted=print.

62. American Diabetes Association. http://www.diabetes.org/about-diabetes.jsp.

63. *New York Times*. "Guide to Knowledge." http://topics.nytimes.com/top/news/health/diseasesconditionsandhealthtopics/bloodpressure/index.html?inline=nyt-classifier.

64. New York City Department of Health and Mental Hygiene. http://www.nyc.gov/health.

65. American Cancer Society. http://www.cancer.org.

66. National Cancer Institute. http://www.cancer.gov.

67. Ibid.

68. The Harvard Center for Cancer Prevention. http://www.yourdiseaserisk.harvard.edu/hccpquiz.pl?lang=english&func=show&quiz=breast&page=fact_sheet.

69. National Cancer Institute, U.S National Institutes of Health. http://www.Cancer.gov.

70. National Institutes of Health. http://www.nhlbi.nih.gov/health/dci/Diseases/Asthma/Asthma_WhatIs.html.

71. Ibid.

72. Food and Nutrition Board, Institute of Medicine, National Academies. *Dietary Reference Intakes: Application in Dietary Planning.* Washington, DC: National Academies Press, 2002.

73. University of Nebraska Cooperative Extension in Lancaster County. "Food Reflections," March 2004. http://lancaster.unl.edu/food/ftmar04.htm.

74. United States Department of Agriculture. "Food and Nutrition Information." http://www.nal.usda.gov/fnic/etext/ds_general.html.

75. *Dietary Guidelines for Americans,* 2005. http://www.healthierus.gov/dietaryguidelines/index.html.

76. Ibid.

77. Ibid.

78. National Heart, Lung, and Blood Institute. *Clinical Guidelines on the Identification, Evaluation, and Treatment of Obesity in Adults: The Evidence Report. NHLBI Obesity Education Initiative Expert Panel on the Identification, Evaluation, and Treatment of Obesity in Adults.* Washington, DC: U.S. Department of Health and Human Services, 1998.

79. American Obesity Association. *Shape Up America! Guidance for the Treatment of Adult Obesity.* Bethesda, MD: Author. Revised 1998.

80. Ibid.

81. National Institute of Diabetes and Digestive and Kidney Diseases. "Gastric Surgery for Severe Obesity." NIH Publication No. 96-4006, April 1996.

82. American Society for Bariatric Surgery. "Rationale for the Surgical Treatment of Obesity." April 6, 1998.

83. Renquist, K. "Obesity Classification." *Obesity Surgery,* Vol. 8, 1998, p. 480.

84. National Institutes of Health. "Consensus Development Conference Statement Online." *Gastrointestinal Surgery for Severe Obesity,* Vol. 1, March 25–27, 1999, pp. 1–20.

85. Kral, J. G. "Surgical Treatment of Obesity." In *Handbook of Obesity,* ed. G. A. Bray, C. Bouchard, and W. P. T. James. New York: Marcel Dekker, Inc., 1998.

86. FDA Talk Paper. "FDA Approves Implanted Stomach Band to Treat Severe Obesity." June 5, 2001.

87. American Society for Bariatric Surgery. "Rationale for the Surgical Treatment of Obesity." April 6, 1998.

88. American Psychiatric Association. *Diagnostic and Statistical Manual for Mental Disorders,* 4th ed. (APA): Washington DC: Author, 1994.

89. Ibid.

90. Hsu, G. L. K. "Epidemiology of the Eating Disorders." *Psychiatric Clinics of North America,* Vol. 19, No. 4, 1996, pp. 681–697.

91. Sullivan, P. F. "Mortality in Anorexia Nervosa." *American Journal of Psychiatry,* Vol. 152, 1995, pp. 1073–1074.

92. Zerbe, K. J. *The Body Betrayed.* Carlsbad, CA: Gurze Books, 1995.

93. American Psychiatric Association, *Diagnostic and Statistical Manual.*

94. Gidwani, G. P., and E. S. Rome. "Eating Disorders." *Clinical Obstetrics and Gynecology*, Vol. 40, No. 3, 1997, pp. 601–615.

95. Kendler, K. S., C. MacLean, M. Neale, R. Kessler, A. Heath, and L. Eaves. "The Genetic Epidemiology of Bulimia Nervosa." *American Journal of Psychiatry*, Vol. 148, 1991, pp. 1627–1637.

96. Zerbe, K. J. *The Body Betrayed.*

97. Smith, D. E., M. D. Marcus, C. E. Lewis, M. Fitzgibbon, and P. Schreiner. "Prevalence of Binge Eating Disorder, Obesity and Depression in a Biracial Cohort of Young Adults." *Annuls of Behavioral Medicine*, Vol. 20, pp. 227–232.

98. Ibid.

99. American Psychiatric Association, *Diagnostic and Statistical Manual.*

100. Ibid.

101. Ibid.

102. Henise, L., M. Ellsberg, and M. Geottemoeller. "Ending Violence Against Women." *Population Reports*, Series L, No. 11, December 1999.

103. National Center for Victim's Crime. http://www.ncvc.org.

104. Bureau of Justice Statistics. "Crime Data Brief, Intimate Partner Violence, 1993–2001." February, 2003.

105. Silverman, Jay G., Anita Raj, Lorelei A. Mucci, and Jeannie E. Hathaway. "Dating Violence Against Adolescent Girls and Associated Substance Use, Unhealthy Weight Control, Sexual Risk Behavior, Pregnancy, and Suicidality." *Journal of the American Medical Association*, Vol. 286, No. 5, 2001.

106. Bureau of Justice Statistics. "Violence Against Women: Estimates from the Redesigned Survey." August 1995.

107. Bureau of Justice Statistics. "Crime Data Brief, Intimate Partner Violence."

108. The National Domestic Violence Hotline. http://www.ndvh.org/educate/what_is_dv.html.

109. Ibid.

110. Ibid.

111. Ibid.

112. L. Walker. *The Battered Woman.* New York: Harper and Row, 1980.

113. Rennison, C. M. U.S. Department of Justice, Bureau of Justice Statistics. "Intimate Partner Violence and Age of the Victim, 1993–99." October 2001.

114. U.S. Department of Justice. "Prevalence, Incidence, and Consequences of Violence Against Women Survey," 1998.

115. Randall, M., and L. Haskell. "Sexual Violence in Women's Lives." *Violence Against Women*, Vol. 1, No. 1, 1995, pp. 6–31.

116. The National Women's Health Information Center. U.S Department of Health and Human Services. Office on Women's Health. http://womenshealth.gov/violence/sexual.cfm.

117. U.S. Department of Health and Human Services. National Institute on Alcohol Abuse and Alcoholism. *Journal: Alcohol Research & Health: Highlights from the Tenth Special Report to Congress, Health Risks and Benefits of Alcohol Consumption* (Volume 24, Number 1, 2000 ed.). Washington, DC: U.S. Government Printing Office. http://www.niaaa.nih.gov/publications/arh24-1/toc24-1.htm.

118. U.S. Department of Health and Human Services. Substance Abuse and Mental Health Services Administration. *Results from the 2001 National Household Survey on Drug Abuse: Volume I. Summary of National Findings* (Office of Applied Studies, NHSDA Series H-17 ed.) (BKD461, SMA 02-3758). Washington, DC: U.S. Government Printing Office, 2002. http://www.oas.samhsa.gov/nhsda/2k1nhsda/vol1/Chapter3.htm.

119. U.S. Department of Health and Human Services. SAMHSA's Center for Substance Abuse Treatment. *You Can Help: A Guide for Caring Adults Working with Young People Experiencing Addiction in the Family* (PHD878, (SMA) 01-3544). Washington, DC: U.S. Government Printing Office. http://www.samhsa.gov/centers/csat/content/intermediaries.

120. Ibid.

121. AMA. http://www.ama-assn.org/ama/pub/category/13246.html.

122. Center on Alcohol Marketing and Youth, January 2006. http://camy.org/factsheets/index.php?FactsheetID=7.

123. Hingson, R., et al. "Magnitude of Alcohol-Related Mortality and Morbidity Among U.S. College Students Ages 18–24: Changes from 1998 to 2001." *Annual Review of Public Health*, Vol. 26, 2005, pp. 259–279.

124. Snyder, L. B., F. F. Milici, M. Slater, H. Sun, and Y. Strizhakova. "Effects of Alcohol Advertising Exposure on Drinking Among Youth." *Archives of Pediatrics and Adolescent Medicine*, Vol. 160, 2006, pp. 18–24.

125. Strasburger, V. C., and E. Donnerstein. "Children, Adolescents, and the Media: Issues and Solutions." *Pediatrics*, Vol. 103, No. 1, 1999, pp. 129–139.

126. Adams Business Media. *Beer Handbook*. Norwalk, CT: Author, 2001.

127. Chura, H., and W. Friedman. "Diageo Moves Forward with Network Plan: Marketer to Run $200 Million in Liquor Ads on TV Consortium." *Advertising Age*, May 13, 2000.

128. Jernigan, D., and P. Wright, eds. *Making News, Changing Policy: Using Media Advocacy to Change Alcohol and Tobacco Policy*. Rockville, MD: Center for Substance Abuse Prevention, 1994; B. Gallegos, *Chasing the Frogs and Camels out of Los Angeles: The Movement to Limit Alcohol and Tobacco Billboards: A Case Study*. San Rafael, CA: The Marin Institute for the Prevention of Alcohol and Other Drug Problems, 1999.

129. J. M. Wallace Jr., et al. "The Epidemiology of Alcohol, Tobacco and Other Drug Use Among Black Youth." *Journal of Studies on Alcohol*, Vol. 60, 1999, pp. 800–809.

130. Substance Abuse and Mental Health Services Administration. *Results from the 2004 National Survey on Drug Use and Health: National Findings*. Rockville, MD: Office of Applied Studies, 2005, table H.25.

131. Centers for Disease Control and Prevention (CDC). "Annual Smoking-Attributable Mortality, Years of Potential Life Lost, and Economic Costs—United States, 1995–1999." *MMWR*. Vol. 51, 2002, pp. 300–303. http://www.cdc.gov/mmwr//preview/mmwrhtml/mm5114a2.htm.

132. American Cancer Society. *Cancer Facts & Figures 2005*. Atlanta, GA: American Cancer Society, 2005.

133. http://www.drugabuse.gov/Infofax/tobacco.html.

134. American Cancer Society, *Cancer Facts & Figures 2005*.

135. Ibid.

136. Ibid.

137. Office of the U.S. Surgeon General. "The Health Consequences of Smoking: Nicotine Addiction: A Report of the Surgeon General, Centers for Disease Control and Prevention (CDC), Office on Smoking and Health. 1988." http://www.cdc.gov/tobacco/sgr/sgr_1988/index.htm.

138. Office of the U.S. Surgeon General. "The Health Benefits of Smoking Cessation: A Report of the Surgeon General, Centers for Disease Control and Prevention (CDC), Office on Smoking and Health. 1990." http://profiles.nlm.nih.gov/NN/B/B/C/T/.

139. U.S. Department of Health and Human Services. Substance Abuse and Mental Health Services Administration. *Understanding Drug Abuse and Addiction: What Science Says: Slide Teaching Packet III, for Health Practitioners, Teachers and Neuroscientists* (AVD145). Washington, DC: U.S. Government Printing Office, 2001. http://www.drugabuse.gov/Teaching3/Teaching.html.

140. U.S. Department of Health and Human Services. Substance Abuse and Mental Health Services Administration. *Summary of Findings from the 2000 National Household Survey on Drug Abuse* (Office of Applied Studies, NHSDA Series H-13 ed.) ([SMA] 01-3549). Washington, DC: U.S. Government Printing Office, 2002. http://www.samhsa.gov/oas/nhsda/2knhsda/chapter2.

141. http://www.drugabuse.gov/Infofax/marijuana.html.

142. U.S. Department of Health and Human Services. SAMHSA's Center for Substance Abuse Prevention. *Prevention Alert: Club Drugs: A New Community Threat* (Volume 3, Number 24 ed.). Washington, DC: U.S. Government Printing Office. http://ncadi.samhsa.gov/govpubs/prevalert/v3i24.aspx.

143. U.S. Department of Health and Human Services. National Institute on Drug Abuse. *NIDA InfoFacts: MDMA (Ecstasy)*. Washington, DC: U.S. Government Printing Office, 2002. http://www.drugabuse.gov/Infofax/ecstasy.html.

144. U.S. Department of Health and Human Services. National Institute on Drug Abuse. *NIDA Info Facts: Rohypnol and GHB*. Washington, DC: U.S. Government Printing Office, 2002. http://www.nida.nih.gov/Infofax/RohypnolGHB.html.

145. U.S. Department of Health and Human Services. SAMHSA's Center for Substance Abuse Prevention. *Prevention Alert: Club Drugs: GHB, an Anabolic Steroid* (Volume 3, Number 27 ed.). Washington, DC: U.S. Government Printing Office. http://ncadi.samhsa.gov/govpubs/prevalert/v3i27.aspx.

146. U.S. Department of Health and Human Services. National Institute on Drug Abuse. *NIDA Research Report: Methamphetamine Abuse and Addiction*. Washington, DC: U.S. Government Printing Office, 2002. http://www.drugabuse.gov/ResearchReports/methamph/methamph2.html#what.

147. http://www.drugabuse.gov/Infofax/methamphetamine.html.

148. Breggin, P. *Talking Back to Ritalin: What Doctors Aren't Telling You About Stimulants for Children*. Monroe, ME: Common Courage Press, 1998.

149. Breggin, P. *Reclaiming Our Children: A Healing Solution for a Nation in Crisis*. Cambridge, MA: Perseus Books, 2000.

150. U.S. Department of Health and Human Services. National Institute on Drug Abuse. *NIDA InfoFacts: Heroin*. Washington, DC: U.S. Government Printing Office, 2002. http://www.drugabuse.gov/Infofax/heroin.html.

151. http://www.drugabuse.gov/Infofax/heroin.html.

152. U.S. Department of Health and Human Services. National Institute on Drug Abuse. *NIDA Research Report—Cocaine Abuse and Addiction* (PHD813, NIH Publication No. 99-4342). Washington, DC: U.S. Government Printing Office, 2002. http://www.drugabuse.gov/ResearchReports/Cocaine/cocaine2.html#what.

153. http://www.drugabuse.gov/Infofax/cocaine.html.

154. U.S. Department of Health and Human Services. National Institute on Drug Abuse. *NIDA InfoFacts: Inhalants*. Washington, DC: U.S. Government Printing Office, 2002. http://www.drugabuse.gov/Infofax/inhalants.html.

155. Centers for Disease Control and Prevention. http://www.cdc.gov/std.

156. Centers for Disease Control and Prevention. "Sexually Transmitted Diseases Treatment Guidelines 2002." *MMWR* Vol. 51, 2002 (no. RR-6).

157. Koutsky, L. A., and N. B. Kiviat. Genital human papillomavirus. In *Sexually Transmitted Diseases*, 3rd ed., K. Holmes, P. Sparling, P. Mardh et al. (eds). New York: McGraw-Hill, 1999, pp. 347–359.

158. American Social Health Association. http://www.ashastd.org.

159. Ibid.

160. Centers for Disease Control and Prevention. *Sexually Transmitted Disease Surveillance, 2002.* Atlanta, GA: U.S. Department of Health and Human Services, September 2003.

161. Holmes, K., P. Mardh, P. Sparling, et al. (eds). *Sexually Transmitted Diseases*, 3rd ed. New York: McGraw-Hill, 1999, chapters 33–37.

162. Centers for Disease Control and Prevention. "Sexually Transmitted Diseases Treatment Guidelines 2002." *MMWR* Vol. 51, 2002. (no. RR-6).

163. Ibid.

164. National Herpes Resource Center and Hotline. American Social Health Association. http://www.ashastd.org/hrc/index.html.

165. Epigee Women's Health. http://www.epigee.org.

166. *New York Times*, Tuesday, January 31, 2006.

167. National Campaign to Prevent Teen Pregnancy analysis of Henshaw, S. K., *U.S. Teenage Pregnancy Statistics*. New York: Alan Guttmacher Institute, 1996.

168. Singh, S., and J. E. Darroch. "Adolescent Pregnancy and Childbearing: Levels and Trends in Developed Countries." *Family Planning Perspectives*, Vol. 32, No. 1, 2000, pp. 14–23.

169. Infectious Diseases Society of America. http://www.idsa.org.

170. National Institute of Allergy and Infectious Diseases. http://www.niaid.nih.gov/publications/microbes.htm#a.

171. Ibid.

172. Ibid.

173. Centers for Disease Control and Prevention, National Center for HIV, STD, and TB Prevention. http://www.cdc.gov/hiv/pubs/faq/faq17.htm.

174. Glynn, M., and P. Rhodes. "Estimated HIV Prevalence in the United States at the End of 2003." National HIV Prevention Conference, June 2005, Atlanta, GA. Abstract 595.

175. *New York Times*, February 4, 2006.

176. AIDS info. http://aidsinfo.nih.gov/.